SLIM BY
THE STARS

June
Baker-Howard

SLIM BY
THE STARS

June
Baker-Howard

RINGPRESS

RINGPRESS

An imprint of Ringpress Ltd.,
Spirella House, Letchworth,
Hertfordshire SG6 4ET

© June Baker-Howard and
Ringpress Books 1990

First published 1990

ISBN No: 0-948955-06-6

Production consultants: Landmark Ltd.
Typeset by Ringpress Books
Printed by Cox and Wyman

CONTENTS

FOREWORD

Astrology is a wonderful aid to self-understanding. It also provides an accurate timing system to tell you when to take action and when to hold back. This awareness is as vital to successful slimming campaign as it is to achieving goals in business or making the right decisions in your personal life.

I have written *Slim By The Stars* to help you use astrology to your advantage; as you become acquainted with the strengths and weaknesses of your sign you will be able to stay more in control of your actions and responses and, therefore, of your weight and figure. By referring to your Astrocharts, you will also know exactly when to begin a diet and, just as importantly, when to guard against over-eating.

Your star sign was determined at the precise moment you were born and it never changes. It represents the *real you*, your potential and the qualities within you.

Here's wishing you every success with your slimming plans.

JUNE BAKER-HOWARD
Spring 1990

HOW TO
USE
THIS BOOK

Once you have read the chapter on your star sign and discovered your own slimming strengths and weaknesses, refer to the Astrocharts for your sign in order to determine your Plus days (indicated by ✓) and your Danger days (indicated by ✗). Plus days occur when the planetary aspects are in your favour . When you begin a slimming campaign, whether it's a short one or a more prolonged effort, be sure always to start it on a Plus day.

Danger days are the days when you may need to take extra precautions against over-eating, so make a note of therm in your diary, or carry this book with you as a reminder. Try to plan your life so that you have plenty to do on Danger days, whether you look to your friends or your hobbies for interesting diversions. Also try to avoid cooking or shopping for food on Danger days The advice on You and Your Emotions and Your Creative Energies will also help you deal with Danger days successfully. Whenever in doubt, re-read your own star sign chapter.

Find the right diet for your astrological personality by turning to the back of this book, where you will find sections headed Air, Earth, Fire and Water. Your sign belongs to one of these four Elements or groups. (For example, Aquarius is an Air sign, and Aquarians will find that an Air diet, started on an Aquarian Plus day will give them the best possible start to a slimming plan.)

Each of these diets has been nutritionally approved and is based on low calorie, low fat eating. The difference between this and other diets is that now you can make use of astrological influences to help you follow the kind of eating pattern that is right for you. And — most importantly — your Astrochart will signal when to start, when to be on your guard, and even when to go back on to your diet if — after a holiday, say — you find that a few pounds have crept back.

Start now, by getting to know yourself. That's the first principal of Slimming by the Stars. After that, your Astrochart and your Element diet — Air, Earth, Fire or Water — will set you, and keep you, on the path to success.

THE STAR SIGN CHAPTERS

ARIES

March 20 - April 19

THE Sun's entry into Aries, around the 21st March, heralds the coming of Spring in the Northern hemisphere. And Aries is the first sign of the zodiac, as well as the cardinal (or principal) Fire sign. There is a strong desire within those born under this sign to initiate action, take control and blaze a trail. Mars, the planet which rules Aries, was called the planet of war by the ancient astrologers, who considered Arians to be especially courageous and bold. The symbol of Aries is The Ram, the assertive leader of the flock.

YOUR SLIMMING PERSONALITY

The key word for your sign, one which sums up your go-ahead personality, is action. An ideal slimming philosophy!

You are a positive thinker and, like the Ram, the symbol of Aries, you tend to tackle life's problems head on. This means that you will soon get to grips with your weight problems.

As a Fire sign, you are quickly motivated and ready to act, but must learn to sustain a steady and constant flame when it comes to dieting, rather than burning yourself out in a sudden bright but short-lived blaze of enthusiastic slimming. Your leadership qualities equip you to inspire others because you capture their imagination with your confident manner and your energy. It is the fiery element within you that urges you to make your mark on the world, and make others aware of your presence.

Even in childhood and throughout your teenage years your tendency to make decisions for yourself, combined with the sheer strength of your will, must have made you a power to be reckoned with. Your ability to take control can at times be misunderstood however, and seen as a sign of rebelliousness or a refusal to accept authority. Muster the force of your will-power now and you will soon lose your surplus weight because there's little that can stand in your way when you have committed yourself to a definite plan of action. Your aim in life should be to make the most of the force of your will, which is a wonderful asset for slimming.

YOUR SLIMMING WEAKNESSES

You prefer to rely on your own experiences rather than those of other people, so you will keep an open mind about your diet plan and Astrocharts until you've tried them for yourself. Learning to have patience and to wait for results is essential to your personal development; this is very necessary if you are to slim successfully, as although you are often the person who initiates new projects, it is easy for you to lose interest if progress is slow, or there is too much boring detail to contend with.

HAVE A SKINFUL
You hate to be kept waiting when you're hungry but there's no need to cook to eat. Dishing up salads and vegetables in the raw, just as nature intended, is especially good for you and none of the nutrients are washed out. Peeling skins off loses vital vitamins — particularly Vitamin C.

One of the root causes of your figure problems could be your hurried life-style. It will assist your slimming efforts if you learn to plan your meals in advance, so you avoid placing yourself in a position where you are suddenly hungry without the appropriate calorie-controlled meal being available. Especially as fast food often consists of fattening and filling snacks, such as french fries and beefburgers — the type of temptation that eases hunger pains but piles on the pounds. Also, never go without food for long periods because you find it difficult to cope with that awful empty feeling, which can cause you to forget your slimming plan.

It's likely that you possess a determined and brave side to your personality. These are the very qualities that can drive you on to success, but can also incline you to take risks or short cuts, that more cautious or less adventurous souls would resist. Be warned, crash diets can reduce your weight in the short term, but tend to add it on with a vengeance in the long-term. This is because your body goes into its survival programme whenever its fuel tanks are depleted, and urges you to increase your intake as quickly as possible, to refill your fatty cells. At the same time, your metabolism slows down, so that you function on less calories than you did originally.

Your desire to see quick results in whatever you start is one of your greatest slimming obstacles because it will be easy for you to become discouraged or impatient if your bathroom scales, or tape measure, fail to come up with the right answers within the expected time-scale.

There is a rebellious side to your nature that doesn't take kindly to too many rules, but to stay slim you must adopt a regular and sensible eating pattern, one which not only provides you with sufficient vitamins and nutrients to deal with the stresses and strains of everyday life, but also leaves you with enough energy to enjoy your leisure time. Insufficient nourishment caused by trying to speed up your weight loss can make you tense, irritable and even difficult to live with. The diet plan given in this book is ideal for your personality.

In your battle against overweight — and this is a battle well worth fighting, both for the sake of your health and also for the pleasure you derive in knowing you look good — you must curb your Aries impatience and only attempt to diet one day at a time.

Complacency can be one of the contributing factors for an Aries weight problem. Sadly, many an Aries has only decided to slim, or taken an active interest in their health, when the damage has already been done.

YOUR SLIMMING STRENGTHS

Where dieting is concerned, you possess a considerable advantage over many of the less decisive signs of the zodiac and those who cannot carry their ideas through. Your spirit, your drive and your willingness to try out something new — all these mean that you are able to grasp the essentials of a dieting routine and make it work for you.

Your speed at forming judgements means that you're unlikely to waste a single day, once you've decided to go ahead. But do consult your Astrochart to check out the most suitable date to begin your slimming plan.

The ambitious, assertive side of

SINFUL SUGAR
Adding sugar to drinks and cereals is strictly forbidden, and one your waistline can do without, so start now to retrain your taste buds. Challenge yourself to stick to the first week of your diets completely sugarless. It becomes easier as you go along and you'll end up hating the sickly sweetness you used to love.

your personality, which likes to win, is one of your slimming strengths. You firmly believe in making your own good luck in life and expect to succeed in whatever you start. You are unlikely to allow others to deter you from your goals and are not over-worried if their eating habits conflict with yours. Indeed you can resent anyone who tries to influence what you put on your plate, or who attempts to impose their likes or dislikes onto you. You also have the strength of character to give up any food that turns out to be injurious to your health or damaging to your figure.

As a decision-maker, you have already confirmed your intention to slim. You have done so by buying this book. Don't be surprised if your friends, colleagues or other members of your household want to copy you by doing something about their own weight or figure problems too. One of your gifts is your convincing way of selling yourself.

BONUS POINTS

You achieve most when you have an incentive to work for. It's possible your parents cashed in on this fact when you were young by offering you sweets or cakes for being good. Cash in now - promise yourself a new outfit or hairdo when you achieve your target weight or a holiday to wear that new slinky swimsuit.

You are ready to work hard to feel proud of your body and can be fairly ruthless with yourself when you discover that your body isn't as slim and supple as it used to be. You like to be in control at all times, especially of your figure and your appetite. In common with other people born under your dynamic sign, you are self-motivated and self-discip-lined, with the will-power to battle on until you are totally satisfied with your overall appearance.

It is your nature to be forthright and get directly to the point of an issue, no matter how painful, so you're not one to fool yourself about your vital statistics, even when the measurements aren't to your liking.

If you're true to your Sun sign, it is important for you to make an impact and show others that you possess a clearly defined sense of identity. Have you noticed how often you like to wear bright, attention-getting colours? This is your way of saying "notice me". It follows that you rarely do go unnoticed - another reason for you to make sure that your image never lets you down.

As it's unnecessary for you to have other people to bolster your confidence, it will not worry you if you have to follow the diets in this book on your own, even if means feeding your family with different meals to keep them happy. In fact, you often prefer to play a lone hand in life and do things in your own sweet way.

You are resourceful and able to cope in times of crisis, so are a wonderful person to turn to in an emergency. This means that you'll be able to point your friends and family in the right direction if they are overweight or if they are experiencing difficulties in following their own diet plan.

You always feel more energetic and ready to take on the world when Mars, your planetary ruler, is passing through your sign, or is in a position in the heavens that is favourable to Aries. These are the times to begin your Astrodiet, or restart it if you've let matters slide. Your "danger days" are when Mars is unfavourably aspected to Aries. You must then put extra thought into keeping yourself occupied and well away from those people who annoy you and could drive you to eating or drinking more than you should. The movements of Mars have been especially taken into account in the calculation of your Astrocharts.

YOU AND YOUR BODY

You are very body conscious. A natural pride in your appearance and keeping fit, means that you are prepared to invest time, money and effort into achieving the weight and the shape that you'd like. It's not surprising that yours is considered to be one of the most energetic signs of the zodiac because your inclination is to take instant action when you are faced with a problem. Although this will get you started on your diet, you must learn to pace yourself. Don't expect too much, too soon.

When you are faced with opposition your instinctive desire is to attack in one form or another. This means that you have to cope with anger and the resultant adrenalin pouring into your blood stream, which can sometimes lead you to eat, or drink, to excess through turning your anger onto yourself and taking

DO-IT-YOURSELF
As you tend to be a do-it-yourselfer, try adding a banana, fresh strawberries or any selection of chopped or puréed fruits, to a carton of plain yogurt, the low-fat variety of course, to make a mouth-watering dessert. You'll enjoy it all the more because you used your imagination and prepared it yourself.

your frustration out on your body. Exercise is an essential part of any slimming plan for you, as you need to find adequate physical outlets for your pent-up energy. Regular exercise keeps you feeling fit and ready to take on the world. Work-outs, weight lifting and activities which allow you to channel any anger, annoyance, aggression or frustration in a healthy way, are ideal. An exercise machine is likely to be the best gift that anyone ever bought you!

Aries people have the reputation for being headstrong, so it's hardly surprising that the head, brain and the eyes are the parts of the body particularly associated with your sign. The symbol of Aries represents the horns of the Ram, another indication that the traits of Aries are recognised as being forceful and insistent, sometimes to the point of being pushy or acting like a battering-ram.

TEMPTATION ON WHEELS
You like to be mobile but resist the temptation to fill up your car with a selection of mints, chocolates, sweets or other 'goodies' in order to combat the boredom of long sessions sitting behind the wheel. It's only too easy for hours spent driving or stuck in frustrating traffic jams, to result in a spare tyre — one of the fatty sort — right round your middle.

Coming to terms with yourself and with the life you have created is part of your recipe for perfect health because your body soon reacts to the way you feel inwardly. When you're unwell, you can usually identify the underlying reason which is often connected with a loss of control in some way, because you are a person who puts great store in staying in control. It is when you feel that your hands are tied, so that you cannot take the action you would like, or you find yourself in a situation where others are issuing the orders, that you are most likely to fall ill or suffer from depression.

YOU AND YOUR EMOTIONS

Whether you realise it or not, you are usually the one who sets the pace in your emotional relationships. Even when you were a small child, it's likely that you made the rules in the playground with your brothers and sisters. Your unwillingness to compromise in life means you will rarely share your time with people who annoy or bore you. You insist on total loyalty from your friends, family and partner and rarely give anyone a second chance if they hurt you, reject you or let you down in any way.

You make an enthusiastic lover or friend, with the potential to fulfil the fiery promise of your sign. What you seek above all, is proof, proof that others love you and need you. You have to be certain of your partner's affections. Because of this, you hesitate to put yourself in the position where you can be snubbed. This means that you sometimes don't put as much effort as you could into cultivating new friendships.

Although you're quite happy in your own company, you like to know that there's a partner waiting in the background, someone who is ready to show you the appreciation which brings out the best in you. You can feel very lonely if you're deprived of company for long periods.

Your reactions are instantaneous, so you're best avoiding moody or unreasonable people. Anger is one emotion that can make you break your diet in a flash. Don't vent your rage by demolishing a plate of sizzling fish and chips or a steaming dish of curry, before you have managed to cool and calm yourself down! It will be too late to consider the damaging implications your upset has had for your figure.

Other people cannot fail to be aware of you and are attracted by your air of confidence. But only diet with someone else if that person is prepared to play a supportive role or is keen to follow your lead. Your feelings are stronger than you sometimes care to admit or show, as you like to put on a brave front at all times. But it's not always easy for you to live up to the dynamic reputation of your Sun sign. Only too often you must find that other people look to you to do their dirty work and make their excuses and complaints, mistaking your brave facade for nerves of steel, not realising that you can be just as unsure of yourself as the next person. When you have achieved your desired weight you are certain to be told by those who don't know you well, that "of course it was easy for you".

You relate particularly well to other Fire signs, Aries like yourself, Leos or Sagittarius. Not only do you benefit from the mutual understanding that exists between all of the Fire people but you are motivated and excited by the competitive element that is sparked off whenever you meet each other, even when you are the best of friends. This competitiveness can provide a tremendous boost in a shared slimming campaign and could be the challenge you need if ever your will-power is in danger of weakening. If there are Water sign people in your life — Cancers, Scorpios or Pisces — beware of their effect on your diet! They are so sensitive that they will "feel for you" and react to your hunger the instant they hear your stomach rumbling. A Water sign will probably urge you to eat — albeit in the name of loving and caring. All Water signs tend to express their affection and friendship by looking after other people, which usually includes offering lashings of food, regardless of whether or not it's really wanted. Unfortunately, rejection of their hospitality can often be taken as a rejection of themselves. You can avoid hurting your Water-partner or friend's feelings however, if you appeal to their natural compassion and understanding. Explain gently just how important it is to you to become slim and healthy and they will soon be helping, instead of hindering you.

Air sign people, Geminis, Libras and Aquarians, will appreciate the reasons behind your desire to lose weight and probably supply you with a long list of additional reasons for dieting. Even so, they'll prefer to let YOU take the plunge and try a diet out first to see how it works and then wait for you to report back to them with the pros and cons before they follow suit. Air and Fire people are very compatible, so usually achieve excellent results when they join forces in a project. The cool, detached objectivity of an Air person helps you to see pitfalls that you could miss in your haste, while in return you give them enthusiasm.

The three Earth signs, Taurus, Virgo and Capricorn could prove to be either your greatest allies or your greatest source of frustration. Their down-to-earth, common sense attitudes will help you to plan and structure your life, so that your imaginative ideas stand more chance of bearing fruit — but conversely, their caution and insistence on taking one step at a time could cause you to miss your moment. Earth people are keenly aware of the importance of food, which they view as a source of pleasure as well as survival. Unless you persuade them to share your diet programme, you'll find your determination is constantly tested by the sight and smell of the tasty food that Earth people know how to prepare. Try to benefit from an Earth person's ability to organise ahead: you could find dieting easier if your meal times are supervised by an Earth-partner or friend.

YOUR CREATIVE ENERGIES

You attack your hobbies with as much enthusiasm as any other area of your life, so often excel in whatever you put your mind to.

Aries tend to walk off with many of the prizes when they enter competitions. However, you're unlikely to compete unless you feel that there's a strong chance of winning because you hate to be second best. Slimming is one competition in which you're guaranteed a prize - if you stick to the rules and follow your diet. In common with the other two Fire signs, Leo and Sagittarius, it's a matter of pride to you to be good at anything you undertake.

In off-duty moments, you like to be busy. You can be tremendously productive, providing you steer clear of projects that drag on for too long or are uninteresting. Your weight-watching will be assisted if you concentrate on those jobs which excite you, so that you don't eat out of boredom.

> **DAWDLING DANGERS**
> *Avoid dining with a Libra, unless you're over-hungry — it could be your undoing. While they are dithering over the menu you will have scooped up bread rolls, olives, nuts or any other appetizers going, in your eagerness to eat. As an impatient Aries, it's not easy for you to wait!*

By using your Astrochart, you will know when you run the risk of over-eating. This will allow you to plan your time accordingly and take preventative measures, such as involving yourself in things that fire your imagination. You're usually most attracted to leisure interests which have a useful side, so often develop a range of skills through the course of your life. Mars, your planetary ruler, is associated with iron and many Aries are adept at working with metal. Engineering and mechanics are typical Aries occupations and even the most feminine Aries tends to be a deft hand with screwdriver and spanner.

Work is one of your prime outlets for creative expression and you put your heart and soul into whatever you do, acting as your own severest judge and critic. The frustration you feel when a job goes wrong, can lead you to finding solace in a snack outside of eating hours. This is a good reason for you to be realistic when assessing the length of time required to complete whatever you've started.

When you feel the urge to take a holiday, your first instinct is to start packing — this can even be before you have actually booked your trip or decided on your destination! Your ideal location has to offer excitement, as you would find it hard to be stranded in a quiet place for too long. A new venue every year would suit your style and love of new adventures. The typical Aries prefers plenty of challenge, lots of bustle and activity. After all, your keyword is ACTION — the reason why you'll make a successful slimmer.

TAURUS

April 20 — May 20

TAURUS, the second sign of the zodiac, is symbolised by the Bull and associated with strength and fertility, indicative of the staying power of those born under this sign. Taurus is ruled by the planet Venus, connected with harmony and beauty. Weather permitting,Venus is clearly visible around the time of sunset, so is often called the Evening Star. As Taurus is the "fixed" (or steadfast) Earth sign, the need for stability and security is a driving force in all Taureans.

YOUR SLIMMING PERSONALITY

Your love of beauty makes you an ideal candidate for slimming as it is particularly distressful to you if your appearance doesn't match up to your own high standards. You are very well aware of the attractive person you can be when your measurements are in proportion to your height because you have a good eye for line and also for colour.

It is natural for you to like good food and wine, because yours is a sign of gracious living and many Taureans are blessed with a hearty appetite, having the ability to eat anything from pickled onions, baked beans, toasted cheese sandwiches, profiteroles and after dinner mints, all at the same meal — without feeling uncomfortable or suffering from the slightest hint of indigestion. Fortunately, slimming doesn't mean that you'll be deprived of all eating pleasures: the diets planned for you in this book allow you to enjoy one or two luxuries and yet lose weight at the same time.

When you plant seeds, they usually flourish because you are gifted with the diligence and the patience to allow them to grow in their own good time. This means that you are able to enjoy the rewards of your labour in every area of your life — and where slimming is concerned, you can use your qualities of perseverance and strength to bring the reward of a new, slimmer and healthier you.

YOUR SLIMMING STRENGTHS

Once you have decided to pursue a certain course of action, you rarely abandon it because you have the great gift of persistence which enables you to work slowly but surely towards your goal. This willingness to apply yourself and stay with your plans is one of your winning attributes when it comes to losing weight.

You are good at organising both yourself and also others, especially children. This means that when you establish a routine, you ensure it can be followed without too much inconvenience or hassle, as your family tends to fit into your own well regulated pattern of living.

> **GROW MORE**
>
> *As Taureans are considered the farmers of the zodiac, it's highly probable that you possess 'green fingers', the hallmark of a good gardener, so why not grow your own salads, tomatoes and other natural produce? The satisfaction of eating home-grown, low calorie and health-giving fresh food that you planted and cared for yourself, even in a window box, will make slimming all the more enjoyable.*

Being practical, determined and sometimes even stubborn is one of your greatest slimming strengths, because you are unlikely to break your diet easily, even if you have a large amount of weight to lose. You are sensible enough to accept that there is no magic formula for slimmers, that the only certain way there is of losing weight and staying slim, is to eat less and take regular exercise.

You tend to prefer set meal times, which can be used to your advantage in your efforts to shed inches, as you can keep a better control on your food intake than those who have erratic eating patterns. Taureans, both men and women, are usually excellent homemakers and housekeepers, so it is natural for you to do the shopping and the planning of meals. However, as you are now preparing to begin a new way of life — a slim, healthy way of life — this is the time to review and rethink your weekly shopping lists.

It will soon become automatic for you to measure your portions before putting food on your plate and so monitor your daily food consumption. It is by retraining yourself to accept new, healthy, slim ways of eating that you'll achieve the shape you'd like to be — and retain it.

Nearly all Taureans have a well developed sense of humour, one of the finest qualities anyone can possess. This ability you have to laugh at yourself, as well as at life generally, is a definite bonus for you as a would-be slimmer. It helps you to see how ridiculous it is to allow the dictates of your stomach to become over-important.

You usually know what you want out of life and can be charming, sweet and persuasive, or blunt, demanding and outspoken, as the occasion demands. A good indication that you have what it takes not only to diet successfully, but to talk others into you way of thinking!

You always feel more at peace with the world and contented with life when Venus, your planetary ruler, is passing through your sign or is in a position in the heavens that is favourable to Taurus. These are the times to begin a new diet, or restart a lapsed one as necessary. Your Danger days are when Venus is unfavourably aspected to your sign. Then you must put extra thought into how you plan your time and try to avoid frustrating situations or loneliness. The movement of Venus has been especially considered in the calculation of your Astrocharts.

YOUR SLIMMING WEAKNESSES

Ideally, you should have been born rich, because you have gourmet tastes. If you can't afford the caviare and champagne lifestyle that you would like, you sometimes try to compensate by awarding yourself generous portions of rich foods.

These may excite your taste buds but unfortunately serve to whet your appetite so that you want even more. As you well know food provides you with the necessary fuel for your body, but any surplus you eat is processed and stored by your body as fat. However unwelcome this fact may be, you can only lose weight by either reducing your calorific intake, or finding a way to increase your output of energy, which almost certainly means a change in your dietary and exercise habits.

SLOWLY DOES IT
Satisfaction can take time to register, so get into the habit of eating slowly. If you're very hungry, eat a small starter to take the edge off your appetite, then wait ten minutes before attacking the main course. If you serve up on a smaller plate than you've been accustomed to, you'll leave the table feeling as if you've had a full size meal.

Your waistline and hips soon suffer if you indulge in too much socialising, so parties, weekends away and holidays pose a formidable threat to your figure. Bliss for you combines luxury and comfort. A love of good food is as natural to you as breathing and many Taureans are tip-top cooks and wonderful hosts and hostesses. This appreciation of the culinary arts and entertaining must be controlled carefully as it is often one of the contributing factors to you putting on weight.

Others tend to turn to you in times of trouble because you possess a certain aura of peace and calm, even when the opposite is the case. Your hospitable nature and kind heart can encourage you to console your loved ones with reassuring plates of comforting food, but as you like to put others at their ease, you often find yourself joining them in eating it — at the expense of your figure.

FREE TO CHOOSE

You need freedom to do your own thing, so your Astrodiet will suit you. As you are allowed to eat more food on some days than others you can swap the whole day's diet plan around if the pattern doesn't match your appetite. If you keep a close watch on what you eat on week days, you can indulge yourself a little at weekends or on special occasions, without worrying too much.

You have staying power and are not easily deterred but when you are confronted with a sudden change in your routine, you are inclined to resist it because you hate upheaval. You do not welcome too much excitement or disruption. You can also be extremely suspicious of anything that's untried and untested. This can make you miss out when progress depends on adapting to new methods. Your reluctance to be adventurous can tie you to traditional but solid eating habits that can gradually make you gain weight, without you being aware of it. That is, until you have a problem. The diet for Earth signs in this book has been carefully adapted with your personality in mind. You will find it easy to comply with once you have accepted the changes that you must make.

YOU AND YOUR BODY

Taureans stand more chance of reaching a ripe old age than any other sign of the zodiac, as statistics show there are an unexpectedly high proportion of those born under the sign of the

Bull amongst the over-eighties. And if you're a typical Taurean, you're blessed with a strong and robust constitution. However, you will probably have to work hard at keeping it in shape, especially as you grow older, because your liking for good food and a comfortable lifestyle are often totally at odds with your body's true requirements.

As the parts of the body associated with Taurus are the neck, throat and chin, your neck is one of your high risk areas for storing fat. You should always keep a careful watch on your chinline and take immediate dieting action if you notice any developing signs of a double-chin.

When taking up exercise, you will find that the gentler forms suit you best, preferably taken at regular times and intervals. Yoga and walking are ideal as they allow you to tone up your body gently and keep it supple without too much effort and discomfort.

Moderation is a key factor in establishing the new you that you're seeking, so plan to exercise every day rather than saving up your good intentions for a grand slam once a week. It's important for you to enjoy exercising and also to know with certainty that the end result will be worth the time and energy you have expended.

Ruled by Venus, associated with the Goddess of love, most Taureans, especially the female members of this sign, are very attractive to the opposite sex.

GETTING ABOUT

As Taurus is considered a 'fixed' or steadfast sign, it's especially essential for you to get up and get moving. Although this diet will work if you stay with it, you will help things along and improve your overall shape by taking excercise every day. Walk, play sport, swim, dig the garden or buy a tape and limber up. But if you join a keep-fit class, beware of those socials!

No doubt you grew from being a bonny, bouncing baby, to a good-looking teenager without giving your luck a second thought. Unfortunately, it is often only after you have allowed your weight to creep up and your figure to lose its ideal shape, that you recognise the necessity for regular weight-watching. Dieting and taking regular exercise are the only way you will be certain of retaining the shapely figure that is rightfully yours. The diets given in this book will make it easy for you to do just this. They also take into account your Taurean appreciation of good food and enjoyment of creative cooking, as well as your liking for entertaining.

It cannot be emphasised too strongly how essential it is for you constantly to keep your eye on your weight and to adjust your daily diet accordingly. This should be a way of life for you if you want to stay slim as, apart from the obvious health risks associated with being overweight, feeling ungainly makes you miserable and lethargic.

YOU AND YOUR EMOTIONS

You're a romantic, chasing ideals and sometimes placing others on a pedestal. To your friends and the ones you love, you are a tower of strength. When you enter into an emotional commitment, you do so with a passion and a conviction that it will last. No power on earth will put you off the one you have chosen. Ideally you need an insurance policy against sustaining emotional hurt because if ever your faith is proved unfounded or misplaced it can be extremely bad news for your figure!

You rarely rush into new relationships because you prefer to get to know people gradually before you allow them into your private and more intimate inner circle. You need to feel comfortable and relaxed with your partner at all times. As you are a person of commitment, you also need someone who reassures you and makes you feel secure, someone you are able to respect and admire. Your Taurean passion can quickly turn to scorn if the object of your affection fails to live up to your expectations and disturbed emotions can produce disturbed eating patterns.

Personal relationships are a serious matter to you because it is essential for you to have harmony in your home and in your leisure time. You are often the hub of the household and usually have ready access to the food store which can be one of your slimming obstacles. You are a fairly resolute character, but remember that your way is not necessarily the only way. Allow the other members of your family or household to have their say

FREEZE WHEEZE
Preparing your own ready-frozen, calorie counted meals will not only save money and time, it will help you change your eating habits and attitudes to what constitutes a sensible meal. Why not batch cook some of your most successful diet-meals — those that work for you because you particularly like them? Then freeze and label them for future use.

in the way things are run, as you may learn a trick or two by paying attention to what they say and watching what they do. Particularly take note of the slimmer members of your household, who are probably naturally following the advice given in this book.

As a friend you are the "salt of the earth" type — staunch, loyal and totally reliable; but you can come unstuck by expecting too much from those you care about, so the ability to accept other people as they are is important for your emotional tranquillity. For you, loving and pleasure go hand in hand because you will shower the person you care about with thoughtful gifts and compliments, as well as good food. Your Astrochart will be particularly helpful to you because it will make you aware of those days when you should take care not to go over the top with edible expressions of your feelings.

Other people love to pin the labels of being "stubborn and possessive" upon Taureans, but you're not as unmovable as some might think. (You can now prove this by successfully completing your diet plan.) Your natural prudence means you will be standing strong when those who jump too hastily have come unstuck. Don't allow your often commendable caution to stop you now, because as a child of the planet Venus, beauty and attraction are your gift by birth-right, a wonderful reason for making the decision to diet.

You are at ease with those born under the other Earth signs, Virgo and Capricorn, as well as other Taureans. However, tread carefully when it comes to eating together, because a common tendency for all Earth people is to equate food with comfort. Even so, Earth people can help to keep you on the right track if they have pledged their support to you. Rely on them to remind you of your "danger days" well in advance. Your attitudes to life and also to eating, are very similar to theirs, so they will understand and sympathise with your problems.

There is usually a natural empathy between you and the Water signs of Cancer, Scorpio and Pisces, who are very sensitive to your needs and to your feelings. Water people can be much stronger and tougher than they appear, so don't hesitate to team up with a Water friend or partner in your slimming campaign — they will help you to keep going. As Water signs are also very sensitive to their own bodies, they can teach you how to tune into your own and make you more aware of the signals your body is constantly sending to you. Most Water people possess a natural gift to heal and soothe others in times of trouble. You can confidently turn to your Water friends when you are feeling tense and so avoid taking your frustrations out on a plate of food.

The intensity and the sheer energy you put into your emotional relationships can be overwhelming for Air people, who value detachment, space and the freedom to come and go as they please. The Air sign individuals you come into contact with, whether they be your close relatives, your partner or your colleagues at work, are certain to approach the whole question of slimming from a different angle to yourself. The reason why they eat can be as much for something to do, as to meet their basic survival needs and energy requirements. Don't expect them to be especially sympathetic to your diet efforts — they are as different to you as chalk is from cheese. The rules and time tables that work so well for you are an anathema to them.

Life should never be dull with a person born under a Fire sign, whether that Fire sign be Aries, Leo or Sagittarius, because their warmth, enthusiasm and ability to enjoy life will stimulate you and encourage you to be adventurous. However, as all Fire signs tend to hold strong views of their own, don't be surprised if you experience an occasional clash of wills between you But they are just what you need to give you a push if ever you're stuck in a rut; and they can motivate you to do something about it instantly if ever your bathroom scales are beginning to creep up past your desired weight limit.

YOUR CREATIVE ENERGIES

Anticipation is a large part of the pleasure you derive from all leisure activities. Like all Earth people, you're good at organising and planning. When you start a project, you expect to see it through, and take pride in your accomplishments. Whether you involve yourself in a business venture or a spare time interest, you spend a long time thinking it through before you start and your eye for detail usually ensures that the end result is perfect — or as perfect as it can be. You are one of the most colour-conscious signs of the zodiac: painting, whether with canvas and easel or paint tin and step ladder, is a wonderful way for you to channel your creative energies. Most Taureans excel at art and interior design and Taureans are well represented in the world of fashion and beauty.

Many famous singers are born under your sign, so it's likely that you adore music and singing. You may possess a good or powerful singing voice yourself. Music stirs your emotions and nourishes your soul. Fortunately, it is harmless to your figure! In fact, it can do you a power of good healthwise if you combine music with dance or exercise .Why not have a sing-song or a knees-up whenever your mind strays to food?

There's a peaceful, quiet side to you, which enjoys curling up with a good book. Apart from reading purely for pleasure, you're also an avid reader of D.I.Y. books as they satisfy the productive side of your personality. Your personal library may well include titles such as How to paint in oils; How to landscape your garden; How to grow bonsai trees; How to crochet, quilt or macrame. And it's a fair bet that cook books occupy a great deal of shelf space in your home. For many Taureans food is a favourite hobby.

DANGER ZONES
Never go shopping for food when you're hungry because the delicous aroma of freshly baked bread or roasted coffee beans can make your stomach turn somersaults. Delicatessens and up-market super-markets are always dang-erous zones for you. Never enter them without arming yourself with a carefully thought-out list Here's an even better idea: why not send someone else out to shop for the weekly groceries?

Pleasant, unhurried and stress-free holidays are a certain passport to delight for you. Time spent in the countryside has special value and meaning to you because being close to nature not only revitalises you but also helps you to feel at peace with the outer world as well as within. You hate hardship, however, so may even choose to go without a summer vacation, rather than settle for leaving the comforts of your own home to stay in accommodation that's not really up to scratch.

There is scarcely a Taurean who doesn't grow plants; bulbs, flowers, cacti, radishes, prize marrows, there's an endless list. You possess a natural empathy with the earth and can usually tap into the life source of the vegetable kingdom, often producing quite magical or beautiful results.

In all these occupations, there is one thing that can stand you in good stead in your campaign to lose weight. You appreciate beauty and are at your happiest where there is harmony. Think of your diet as a steady road to a beautifully proportioned you — and to a flowering of your inner personality.

GEMINI

May 21 — June 20

GEMINI, the third sign of the zodiac, represents the transition of spring-time to summer in the northern hemisphere. Ruled by Mercury, the closest planet to the Sun and also the fastest moving planet in our zodiac. Gemini is the mutable (or moving) Air sign and the urge to communicate is a driving force in those born under this sign. In the heavens, the constellation of Gemini is noticeable by two very bright stars, Pollux and Caster. Hence the idea that Gemini is a dual sign. This duality is also indicated by the glyph of the sign, the Roman numeral II — representing the two sides of the Geminian personality, male and female, extrovert and introvert.

YOUR SLIMMING CHARACTER

There are two distinct sides to your personality and to slim successfully you must learn to cater for both.

The opposing elements within you often urge you to try to "have your cake and eat it", and sometimes you manage to succeed in doing so. But not when it comes to dieting, as your figure soon reminds you.

There is a friendly, extrovert and active you and a quiet and more passive you as well. You are not brazen, but you are not shy either.

Life usually forces you into situations where you have to learn to choose wisely. Until you do so, you rarely find peace of mind. Your choice of food influences whether you are slim and dynamic, or sluggish and overweight, so this particular choice is an easy one for you to make, as no Gemini ever likes to look older than their years.

Like the wind you need to be free to come and go as you please, so it is likely that you are quick in both thought and action and find yourself constantly on the move. If you are a true Gemini, you are eager to live your life to the full and extend the summer-time of your life as long as possible, often refusing to accept the idea that you can ever grow old. Your desire to enjoy many different experiences has earned your sign a label: the "butterfly of the zodiac". You like variety — to flit from one activity to another — and this is your key to successful dieting.

Quick-silver, a liquid metal which possesses the property of responding instantly to changes in temperature, is also called Mercury and it is to be expected that your temperament, as a Gemini and one of Mercury's children, should also reflect this ability to react in a flash to external stimulus. You are the kind of person who tends to take on more than one thing at a time, changing your activity to suit your mood. Follow the diets given in this book with confidence because they been created with this liking for flexibility in mind.

YOUR SLIMMING STRENGTHS

A heartening thought for you is that Gemini is essentially a "slim" sign and also a youthful one. Many Geminis look and act much younger than their years, with a lightness of step and a brightness of eye that makes the Gemini man, or woman, whatever their age, an attractive and vital person. The problem of overweight is in fact an uncommon one for Geminis, as your restless energy provides you with the means of staying slim and retaining a youthful figure. This knowledge should encourage you to stick to your diet, because once you have succeeded in your slimming campaign and reached your target weight, your own zodiac temperament, combined with your new self-awareness, should see to it that you remain slim, with only the occasional need to watch your eating habits.

SLIMMING-TALK
Talking, which is your main mode of self-expression, is a wonderful aid to weight watching, so pick up the phone when you're hungry. Your disposition particularly likes a sounding board - someone who gives you a feedback on how they think you're doing and, as a socially aware Gemini, you are sure to be polite enough not to talk with your mouth full!

Geminis are ruled by their minds rather than their emotions, so it follows that once you have talked yourself into taking positive action to resolve your overweight problem, you are already half-way towards achieving success. In fact, your mind needs to be supplied with a constant supply of food for thought. Fortunately, this is better for your slimming plan than providing too much food for your body. You rationalise and analyse carefully every scrap of information that is presented to you, so will appreciate the medical reasons as well as the cosmetic ones for retaining a healthy weight.

You are attracted by a wide range of interests. This can be used to your advantage now as you have the ability to find plenty of worthwhile distractions in order to take your mind off food. A perpetual interest in what's new, novel, the current vogue or out-of-the-ordinary means that you will be ahead of others in trying out your diet plan. At the same time you'll enjoy talking about it to your friends.

If you're typical of your sign, your mind is an active one, with a natural curiosity in anything and everything. Even as a child you probably exhausted your parents and teachers with questions beginning with "Why", "How", "What" and "When". This "child-like" inquisitiveness is likely to continue throughout your life and represents a natural strength where slimming's concerned. Your healthy interest in what's happening in the world at large and in what motivates other people and makes them tick, not only helps you to stay young, but also allows you to switch your mind off the sort of problems that drive those who are more pedestrian in their way of thinking to seek their answers in food and drink.

Your great gift of versatility can be utilised to assist you in reducing your weight: you can combine dieting and exercise and still fit in the thousand and one jobs and activities that you usually have on the go, without any of them suffering. Your love of being active makes staying fit especially desirable, because aches, pains and bodily twinges are rarely your favourite topic of conversation.

When you commit yourself to a project, you expect it to work, and to work quickly. You live for the moment, rather than the past, or the future, so you want to see results NOW!, TODAY! and IMMEDIATELY! You will appreciate the fact that you can throw yourself into your slimming campaign knowing with certainty that you will soon be enjoying the slimmer you. As

MASTERMINDING

You find it easier to stay slim when you are involved in a project which stretches your mind, so swotting up on politics, antiques, the weather patterns, health matters or the balance of payments all helps to keep the pointer on your bathroom scales from zooming up.

you begin your diet you will have taken a very definite and important step towards regaining that slim and fit look that is the true reflection of the inner you. A wonderful incentive for you: begin now to sort out and plan your food cupboards ready to start your diet with a flourish on the exact date given in your Astrochart.

YOUR SLIMMING WEAKNESSES

You collect people with as much enthusiasm as schoolboys put into collecting postage stamps or football programmes. This means that over the years, your circle of friends is inclined to increase rather than diminish. You are at your best when you are in one of your frequent sociable moods surrounded by an appreciative audience. You rarely pass by an opportunity to socialise, especially if it provides the chance to go somewhere new. Here lies your greatest slimming weakness, as eating out is often detrimental to your figure.

EGGSTACY
Ever tried a cold omelette? It makes a surpisingly substantial meal. On days when you are allowed eggs on your diet, make one with your low-fat spread allowance and let it go cold. You could vary this theme by adding a selection of any vegetables that the Air sign diet allows. Alternatively, you can serve it up with a salad.

Another slimming hazard, so far as you're concerned, is your healthy interest in anything new or different. Ironically, this could, if channelled wisely, become one of your greatest slimming strengths. It is essential to be aware of the negative side of your readiness to experiment. Unusual recipes, such as foreign cuisine, can prove irresistible to you as you are usually game to try anything, such as a spicy pizza or well-filled vol-au-vent, at least once. The risk to your figure is twice as high if what you're sampling has the makings of a entertaining talking point.

As already mentioned, Gemini is a mutable — or moving — Air sign, so it is usual for you to be on the move. As a busy, active person, it's essential for you to swot up on the foods allowed in your diet as well as the quantities permissible. Eating too many quick snacks, which are often very high in calories, or deficient in nutrition, is another of your slimming obstacles because when you find yourself under pressure or dashing about from one place to another, it's only too easy for you to grab an instant snack, one that's readily available. In fact, it is the small nibbles that represent your Achilles heel.

It's highly probable that you sometimes start to nibble purely because for the reason that you lack something to do which holds your interest. Finding enough mental stimulus is all-important for you if you are to avoid eating out of restlessness and frustration, so plan to change your surroundings and vary your routine whenever you detect any early warning signs of boredom. Whenever you're tempted to occupy your mind with thoughts of food in between meals, change the subject. Turn on the television, read a good book, start decorating your lounge or go somewhere where there's no food to hand. Even better, begin an exercise session, as this will keep both your mind and body busy working towards a profitable goal — your desired shape and figure. Mini-snacks are permitted only if they are taken from your daily diet as given in this book.

YOU AND YOUR BODY

The hands, the arms and the nervous system are the parts of the body particularly associated with Gemini. No doubt you gesticulate or "talk" with your hands, which are rarely still. You find it stressful if you are forced to stay immobile for long periods and in fact rarely sit still for long in your everyday life. When you take exercise, it should be of the fun variety, easy to do and sociable in nature, preferably of the type that can be done out of doors in the fresh air. Cycling, dancing, gardening and keep fit classes are all likely to appeal to your healthy desire to stay active. Team up with like-minded friends to take exercise and you'll find it twice as rewarding because you will also be able to satisfy your liking for congenial company.

Even so, do allow adequate time for your more serious, introverted side, as periods of peace and quiet are essential for you. These must be balanced with those of a more lively nature to ensure that you

PICTURE PROOF
When you've slimmed right down to your target size, ask a friend to take a photograph of you — then keep it with you wherever you go. Look at it every time you sit down to eat, just to remind yourself what you stand to lose if you over-indulge. All the foods in your Astrodiet are calorie-kind to you and nutritious.

stay in good spirits and in harmony with yourself. Your conflicting needs should never be ignored because being aware of your own complex personality is an important part of your personal healthy living programme. On the one hand, too much exposure to hustle and bustle and too many claims on your resources exhausts you, so that you lose your sparkle and "joie de vivre", while on the other, too much solitude and lack of stimulus depresses you and drags you down.

It is your abundant enthusiasm for both work and play that keeps you young at heart, so it follows that your appearance should reflect the exuberant inner you — the you that is slim, attractive and eternally youthful. It is not easy for you to accept that you're overweight, as it rarely feels natural to you for your body to be too fat or out of shape.

Regular exercise is essential to you and does wonders for your state of mind and confidence as well as your circulation, muscle tone and overall shape. Stretching your body and limbering up helps you to combat stress and mental fatigue as well as keeping you slim and supple. This is an important point to remember because your lively restlessness can sometimes take its toll on your nervous system.

GET YOUR OATS
Look out for a new generation of breakfast cereals based on oats, which provide a healthy alternative to muesli and bran as listed in your Astrodiet. It's important to avoid sugar-coated or sweetened cereals, but if you really miss sugar on them, try a sprinkling of dried fruit instead.

Having adequate rest periods and correctly balanced meals are vital if you are to feel in peak condition, so establishing a good set of habits is very important for your health and body care. A splendid tip for healthy living is to give yourself regular breaks between tasks. Ten minutes relaxation before you charge off on a new assignment could do you more good than many a tonic that comes out of a bottle. Your innermost urge is to communicate, so your body language is usually fairly expressive — all the more reason to look after your body and make sure that it doesn't give the wrong messages due to being overweight or out of breath.

YOU AND YOUR EMOTIONS

Flirting is traditionally considered to be a favourite pastime for a Geminian. Whether or not this is one of your pleasures, there is no doubt that those born under the sign of Gemini do hold a great deal of sex appeal. All the more reason for you to keep a regular check on your weight. You are exhilarated by the glamour and excitement of an initial attraction but may have some lessons to learn about handling and sustaining a long-term relationship.

You seek a lively, versatile and resourceful partner, one who is well-informed and on your wave length. He or she should also be as intelligent as you because you soon become bored with people who are dull or have little to say for themselves. However as you tend to keep the various parts of your life in separate compartments, you can sometimes fail to give your most important personal relationships as much time and attention as you should, or could. It's imperative not to neglect your romantic side: try thinking about the one you love, and planning happy moments together — it's a better aphrodisiac for you than anything that you can eat or drink!

You are a thinker who is inclined to live in your head and often find it difficult to keep your mind off any problems that have become urgent or are likely to arise in the near future. Generally, you prefer to stay in control of your moods and feelings at all times — and you like other people to do the same. This means that you usually try to avoid anyone who makes too many emotional demands, especially as you find it hard to cope with heavy, intense scenes or floods of tears.

Even so, you are fatally attracted to the sensitive Water sign people, Cancers, Scorpios and Pisces because they have what you lack: a natural awareness of their own feelings and emotions, which you sometimes suppress. You are opposites in every way. You form judgements by using reason and logic: Water signs do so through their impressions and feelings. You are analytical and detached — they tend to accept life at face value and be subjective. (Nothing can infuriate you more than a Water sign person's ability to come up with the right answers for what you consider to be the wrong reasons!) If you are trying to diet, don't let a Water sign invite you for a meal — they'll take your refusal of food as a personal rejection — and you know how you hate a scene! Better to enlist their sympathy and support by explaining beforehand.

Geminis, in common with other Air sign people, Librans and Aquarians, must have space and opportunities to develop their own interests and freedom of movement. A relationship with any one of these signs stands a good chance of working out for you because your needs are similar. An Air partner or friend will respect your desire for privacy and will also be in tune with you mentally. Like you they will arrive at conclusions by thinking things through in a logical sequence, refusing to be influenced by emotional or sentimental arguments. Slimming with an Air partner will prove mutually beneficial to you both because you'll be able to talk each other through the Danger days and keep dieting and food matters in perspective.

Aries, Leo and Sagittarius, the three Fire signs, are extremely compatible with Gemini. Fire people inspire you with their flair and their boldness. You can usually spot any flaws in their imaginative ideas and help them to succeed. However, their bluntness can sometimes offend you. This trait can be useful for your slimming attempts as you can count on honesty if you ask for their opinion of your problem areas. They have an uncanny knack of getting straight to the root cause of a matter.

Earth people, those born under Taurus, Virgo and Capricorn, deal with realities, while you deal with possibilities and probabilities. They call a spade a spade and fat FAT, while you prefer to examine the reasons WHY you've added inches, and consider the cause as important as the effect. A close relationship with an Earth person can help you put structure into your arguments. At the same time you can encourage them to be more flexible in their way of thinking. You'll impress an Earth partner or friend most by showing them that you too can wait for results. As they believe in facts rather than speculation tell them to keep watching your figure as every day of your diet is another day closer to your target weight.

YOUR CREATIVE ENERGIES

You are happiest with a series of hobbies because your desire to learn is one of your greatest motivations. Evening class, discussion groups, workshops, books and the whole range of practical and scientific programmes offered through television, videos and films are tailor-made for Geminis.

You are a communicator who takes in information and passes it on in one form or another: if you join a reputable slimming club, you will soon be happily swapping slimming tips and encouraging others to follow your good example. Your instinctive nervous reactions tend to be quick and although you may be agile and good at working with your hands — painting, writing, sewing, knitting, upholstery, hairdressing — you are usually better off at mental pursuits than heavy physical tasks. You stand more chance of being happy and therefore healthy and slim if your occupation and your lifestyle allows you freedom of movement.

The company of convivial friends is as vital to your well-being as the air that you breathe and if you're typical of your airy sign, you find that striking up new acquaintances and relationships comes easily to you. Your ease with words and ready wit equips you to teach, sell and handle others confidently. Make sure that you are as poised and confident as you appear by being proud of your figure. The outward-going side of you is the one that most impresses others. It is because of this, that yours is considered to be one of the most friendly and gregarious

DEEP WATERS
Stay clear of casual Earth sign acquaintances, Taurus, Virgo or Capricorn, on your Danger days. Their self-containment can make you feel inadequate or superficial, so that you seek solace in food. A challenge will do you more good, so seek out the company of a mysterious Water sign person: a Cancer, Scorpio or Pisces.

signs of the zodiac. Anything new, novel or different appeals to you, so when you choose a venue for a special night out, it is likely to be the latest play, eating place or disco. Bright lights and plenty of action suit the bill, particularly if they will provide plenty of material for future discussions. Dinner parties, cabarets, pantomimes, any function that provides interesting personalities and stimulation — these are all for you. Any excuse to meet up with your friends is enough to set you organising drinks, snacks, suppers or tea and biscuits. Your Gemini willingness to sit and chat can pose a problem if you're dieting as you may find that you're nibbling your way through the afternoon or the evening.

Bringing people together is one of your greatest delights, especially if they are unlikely to meet each other in their normal social spheres. It's probable you attract a varied selection of people to your side as there is nothing you enjoy more than listening to different points of view, in fact the more unusual or controversial the conversation the better. Divide the time you spend on leisure activities between those projects you can do on your own and those which involve other people as you will then satisfy the two different sides of yourself — as two people you can expect to be twice as pleased once you have achieved your target weight.

CANCER

June 21 — July 22

THE MOON rules Cancer. The Moon controls the tides and there does seem to be an ebb and flow to the Cancerian personality. Cancerians have an inbuilt calendar which follows the Moon's phases, so they alternate between periods of feeling extremely outward going and periods when they tend to be withdrawn and want peace and quiet. Although the sign of Cancer is the cardinal (or principal) Water sign, it happens to be the least conspicuous sign of the zodiac. The symbol of Cancer is the Crab, and like a crab Cancerians tend to make their home their haven. Also in keeping with the crab, Cancerians possess an extremely soft, vulnerable side to their nature, which they sometimes hide under a thick defensive shell.

YOUR SLIMMING CHARACTER

Your first slimming task is to learn to say "No" when others offer you food. Not because you're a greedy person — Cancer is not a particularly self-indulgent sign — but because you are reluctant to hurt someone else's feelings. Ask yourself this question. As a child, did you try hard to eat up all the food you were given, even if you weren't hungry, just to please your mother or those who cared for you? The answer is almost certain to be "Yes" because as a Cancerian you're extremely sensitive to others. Even now, when you're eating with your friends, family or partner, you may find it difficult to wave away the dessert or second helping of a delicious meal that has been cooked especially for you. You often have strong feelings of guilt when you need to turn down someone else's gesture of love or friendship. This Cancerian trait of saying "Yes" to please others makes it easy for you to put on unwanted pounds and inches when you're sharing food and drink with those you like or care about. The more sociable and friendly the mood, the greater the risk to your figure.

YOUR SLIMMING WEAKNESSES

It's not for nothing that Cancer is considered the sign of the World Mother. Your ability to find fulfilment in life revolves around looking after others, belonging to a unit and "mothering" the people you care about.

Here rests your greatest problem, so far as slimming is concerned. The satisfaction you feel from sharing food you've lovingly prepared for your family or guests can quickly undo all the good work of a week's hard dieting. And your figure is equally at risk when you accept hospitality, especially when the person who presses you to "just have another drink" or "just finish this last slice" is a loving friend or relative. Your key to success lies in understanding this side of your nature.

BE ANTI-SOCIAL TO SLIM
You are a wonderful hostess but your dinners, or parties, can sometimes lead to your own un-doing! It's best not to entertain when you're on a diet, unless you can adapt a diet meal to suit your guests. Try to keep your portions controlled. Never put temptation in your own way by preparing high-calorie foods.

That word "Mother", so frequently associated with your sign, sums up your strong urge to nourish, nurture and care for the other people in your life. Your first instinct, when someone enters your home, is likely to be to feed them, whether you do so by offering them a cup of tea or coffee and a biscuit or a full-scale meal.

But there is a flip side to this mothering urge. The truth is that you also find it very hard to resist when someone wants to mother and look after *you*. This is when you find it hard to say "No". Any concern shown for your well-being is usually warmly received on your part. This is because you delight in being pampered and fussed over. Deep down in the recesses of your subconscious mind, you equate caring with security and are reminded of the safety, warmth, love and attachment of your early years, or of the loving care you missed out on and have searched for all your life.

You can cope with an unlimited supply of love, so if love and affection are being offered to you in the form of food and nourishment, it isn't easy for you to refuse. This means you sometimes accept meals or drinks when you're not really hungry. Apart from any other consideration, your natural sensitivity and understanding of others means that it is not your way to offend your prospective host or hostess by rejecting the gesture of goodwill and friendship that has been kindly offered.

YOUR SLIMMING STRENGTHS

You can use your Cancerian sensitivity to work out the best way to refuse without offending others. A white lie, such as "I had a big breakfast/I ate earlier/I couldn't manage another mouthful" may be easier than explaining that you are trying to lose weight if you are at the kind of gathering where well-meaning friends might see your diet as unnecessary. With closer family and friends, enlist their help and support. You'll experience the feelings of love and security that are so important to you if you have others on your side, helping you towards your goal.

Nevertheless, you may have to eat alone for at least one meal each day. As you probably know only too well, the cooking of an attractive and satisfying meal for your family, or the one who matters most in your life, is often your favourite (and sometimes most fattening) way of expressing your love. You rarely enjoy eating alone, so turn this to your advantage if you are eager to make headway in your slimming campaign .

Your greatest advantage is your wonderful Cancerian quality of tenacity. You rarely give up once you have set your sights on a target. Your tremendous persistence can carry you through when other would-be slimmers are giving up. Use this gift of tenacity throughout your slimming campaign and you will achieve your desired weight and shape. Even if you hit a time when you consider you are failing in your diet, call upon that tenacity and try and try again, because you're sure to win in the

WEIGH UP TO WIN

Cancerians often love to cook but must remember that portion control CAN'T be done by guess-work. Do buy a set of scales, on which you can measure precise ounces, half-ounces and even quarter-ounces, as well as their metric equivalent. Keep on using them until you can recognise the right amount of food without error. Buy a set of measuring spoons too — these will help you to save calories as you cook.

end. Make no mistake: you are capable of achieving the goal you set yourself. Your sign is famous for its ability to "hang on" no matter what it takes.

Another advantage of your sign is your special sensitivity to the twenty-nine day lunar cycles. These are taken into consideration in your Astrochart.. Keep a note of the dates of the New and Full Moons each month, because they are particularly important to you when you are dieting — also when you are following any kind of keep-fit regime.

The day of the Full Moon and the day that follows it are always the best days of any month for you to begin any new diet, or to start again if you've failed to stick to a diet.

Your chances of losing surplus pounds quickly are then at a peak. (You should also choose the time around the Full Moon to discard any other unwanted behaviour pattern, such as smoking.) You may notice that you feel especially dynamic and optimistic when the Moon is waxing — that is during the days leading up to the Full Moon — so this is another excellent indication that you will be able to make a good start with your slimming plan, and stay with it. Choose the time around a

BE PREPARED

Preparing meals for the family can be a tempting exercise for you, so try to organise your time so that you can deal with this task when you've just eaten. That way, you won't want to nibble what you're making. Wrap and refrigerate or freeze food until it's wanted and you'll be far less tempted to pick at it.

New Moon to start an exercise programme or take up a new energetic hobby.

It's likely that you feel more lethargic and unsettled at this time of the month, so will benefit from taking up a new interest, especially if it channels any pent-up energy into a worthwhile goal. When using your Astrochart, take special note of the Danger days when dieting will be difficult, and avoid situations which could set you back in your diet campaign.

Try to arrange any social functions you wish to host or attend on Plus Days, when your willpower will help you withstand the temptations that could arise.

When planning your meals for a week, choose Plus days for those very ambitious culinary efforts and Danger days for less complicated meals, so that you can stick to a safe and structured way of eating.

YOU AND YOUR BODY

As a Cancerian you are especially sensitive to the messages your body sends to your brain, even if you sometimes choose to ignore what they are telling you.

To prove the point, open the door of your refrigerator or food cupboard and imagine eating one of the items to see how your body responds. Work through the possible snacks you can have and ask your body which it prefers. You could be surprised at the result. A craving for a particular food can indicate the necessity to top up on essential vitamins or minerals.

You are usually acutely conscious of the effect that over-eating, drinking, smoking or neglecting to exercise regularly has on your health and your shape. The parts of the body associated with Cancerians are the midriff, waist and breasts. These are your most vulnerable areas for storing surplus fat.

> **NIFTY NIBBLING**
> *If you want to eat between meals, be clever by dipping into your next meal in advance, rather than eating extra bits and pieces. A slice of fruit, or a mouthful of fresh, raw salad vegetables, will appease any hunger pangs and keep you on the straight and narrow, diet-wise.*

You should favour the kind of exercise that is enjoyable rather than hard work. If you can rope in a friend to join you, so much the better. Cancerians are usually particularly happy when swimming, sailing, dancing or doing any kind of exercise that combines movement with music.

The saying "prevention is better than cure" is particularly true in your case, because the sight of your own naked body in the mirror, if it is bulging in all the wrong places, can upset you for the day. You can be your own severest critic when it comes to your appearance. Keeping a constant eye on your weight and vital statistics is your best strategy to stay slim because the prospect of having to pare off large amounts of excess weight is especially hard for a sensitive Cancerian to bear. Make up your mind always to take immediate action — after consulting your Astrochart — if the pointer on your bathroom scales creeps round to your personal danger level.

As far as your general health is concerned, your personality type is an important factor in your predisposition to certain types of illness, and a key factor in your approach to eating. It is by understanding yourself that you will begin to see why you're the weight and shape you are. Sometimes changes must occur within ourselves before we can get to grips with the changes we would like in our outward appearance.

It cannot be emphasised enough that knowing yourself is an important part of maintaining a healthy body and a positive outlook on life. Learning to acquire an inner state of calm is vital for you to stay healthy, happy and slim. Constant stress or anxiety takes its toll on your nervous system and digestion and will eventually leave its mark on the way you look. It is essential to include clearly defined periods of rest in your programme, even if that means turning a blind eye to the mountain of jobs which you are always well aware of.

YOU AND YOUR EMOTIONS

You long to be liked as well as loved. Your instinctive reaction is to put others first, which can make you neglect your own needs and interests. Cancer is the leading, or Cardinal, Water sign. The element of water is associated with sensitivity, feeling and emotions. With you, feelings and emotions always run deep, and this is true whether those feelings are usually calm and peaceful or turbulent and overwhelming. Unfortunately, this means that your eating patterns can soon be disrupted if you are upset or worried. You can alternate between completely losing your appetite through feeling "choked up", to miserably eating your way through a bout of depression regardless of the consequence in terms of unwanted inches or pounds. For these reasons it is important for you to learn to control your eating patterns when your emotions get out of hand.

> **TENDER TRAPS**
> *Your friends pose the greatest threat to your diet intentions. Beware a Leo's love of pampering others and keep a firm eye on your waistline if dining with Taureans, who are often super cooks. Be extra-careful to have eaten, or have your own meal prepared, before feeding an impatient Aries, as fast food tends to be fattening.*

Have you noticed that you sometimes have an inclination to take things too personally? This over-sensitivity to criticism can cause you unnecessary pain and can even be the underlying reason for any health problems you may experience. Your best way to cope when facing criticism is to learn to stand back a little and become an observer of life, rather than becoming too involved in every issue.

The ability to detach yourself — to stand back — will go a long way to giving you the peace of mind that you need in order to overcome the urge to eat or drink when you are feeling in need of comfort.

Also, because of your great need for affection (and because yours is an especially romantic sign) you also need to know how to adjust your slimming efforts so that they fit in with your relationships.

This will be easiest if your closest friends, family and loved ones are also Water signs like you. The other Water signs — Scorpio and Pisces — share your sensitivity, and you may even find that their weight fluctuates as yours does. It will be ideal, of course, if you can persuade a fellow Water sign to follow the diet along with you. But if your partner, although a Water sign, does not need to slim, you should persuade him (or her) to read this book so as to be able to understand your Plus Days and Danger Days. You can rely on a fellow Water sign to understand your moods, and to share your triumphs and elation. Don't be shy, either, about turning to a Water sign for sympathy on days when you feel that the going is tough.

You can gain comfort, too, from a partner who is an Earth sign — Taurus, Virgo or Capricorn. But in this case you will be benefiting not from their sensitivity but from their "down to earth" approach. Don't be offended if you find that your Earth sign partner or friend tries to cheer you up by offering food or drink (the last thing you need) as comfort. Just explain: "I know you mean well, but I shall feel bad if I don't stick to my plan". Earth signs appreciate ambition and determination — even stubbornness — and will like and respect you all the more.

If there are Air sign personalities if your life — friends, partners, close relatives — you will know that this strong mutual attraction is one that allows room for both stimulating conversation and also argument! Those born under Gemini, Libra and Aquarius like to debate and discuss, and may at times be inclined to undermine your confidence in your diet by suggesting other, alternative, ways to slim — or even tell you it's all in the mind and that you do not need to slim at all. Your best way to deal with them without upsetting yourself is to stay calm and appeal to their reason. Say something like: "I understand your point of view, but this is something I want to try for myself". Air signs admire independence, but hate emotional outbursts. If you show them this book you may even help them to learn to be more like you, able to tune into their own innermost feelings.

Perhaps the most challenging of relationships for a Cancerian is that which exists with any of the Fire Signs: Aries, Leo and Sagittarius. You can sometimes find that their energetic and assertive approach to life is almost overwhelming. Nevertheless, it is this very energy and self-confidence that could be the greatest support you need, if you can enlist the help of a Fire sign when dieting. A Fire sign friend or partner who also needs to lose weight could be a tremendous ally — and add a competitive note to proceedings. Follow your individual diets together, even join a slimming club together, and your relationship could blossom, because the qualities of the Fire sign could help you to overcome inhibitions and make you believe in your own ability to stay slim and achieve the shape you've set your sights on.

YOUR CREATIVE ENERGIES

Your slimming programme will be helped by finding time for diversions and activities that keep you pleasurably occupied — and stop you thinking about food. With this in mind, you should plan to indulge in the hobbies, and even the holidays, that are right for your sign.

Although the popular myth of Cancerians is one of domesticity, you demand far more from life that washing dishes and doing domestic repairs. It is essential for you to have an absorbing interest, independent of other people. Unlike many other signs of the Zodiac, you are quite capable of keeping more than one project on the go at a time, knowing they all stand a good chance of being completed.

Cancer is a very creative sign, so you may be good at many different forms of creative expression. Cooking, decorating, gardening, interior design, dressmaking, hairdressing, wine-making...there's an almost endless list of home crafts you can turn your hand to. You can also do well in other creative pursuits and many Cancerians are inspired writers, poets, musicians and artists. This is because your deep feelings pour into your work and add a meaningful content to it.

Your inspiration tends to be at a high when you are happy and full of the joys of life. When you feel a creative mood coming on, you should try to take advantage of it, as not only does it give you intense satisfaction to produce a tangible result from your imagination, but any thoughts you have of nibbling food or of sipping drinks disappear like magic when you are keen to finish a project you've started.

This ability, which you share with two other Water signs, Scorpio and Pisces, to immerse yourself in whatever you are doing, is one of your greatest assets when it comes to watching your weight. In fact, your antidote to over-eating could be to throw yourself wholeheartedly into a new interest. The hours will then slip by unnoticed before someone else's demands for food, or your own sheer hunger, remind you that it's time to eat.

> **MOVE IT!**
> *Look on being active as an important part of keeping your weight under control, as you're more likely to stick to your diet if you've plenty to do. Resist any tendency to brood on life, when you should be getting out and enjoying it more. Get up, get out and get moving. You'll feel better for it.*

You can usually keep yourself occupied and may take your leisure activities extremely seriously. Many Cancerians earn money from their hobbies, either by establishing a profitable sideline, or by turning a favourite hobby into a career or business.

You enjoy being organised by someone else, providing they do it efficiently. Indeed you admire those who exhibit good organising skills, especially if they combine them with imagination. For this reason you could be a good candidate as a member of a recognised slimming club that places an emphasis on sensible eating. You should consult your Astrochart as to the best date on which to join such a club. If however you are, like some Cancerians, too shy or retiring to be a "joiner", don't despair — your qualities of determination are more than enough to enable you to achieve your goals on your own.

Cancer is one of the four Cardinal Signs — which means you are happiest when you are active. Your perfect holiday must include something to do, other than just lazing around, especially as holidays are one of the most hazardous times for your figure, when moments of boredom encourage you to over-eat. Being near, or on, the water soothes and heals you, whether you are strolling along a river bank or sailing on the sea.

Whatever activity you plan, whatever your way of life, you will soon discover that your Astrochart, combined with your special

Water sign diet, is an invaluable aid to keeping yourself shipshape. It will have you streamlining your figure while more sceptical friends are still dithering. Look up your best date to start this month. Remember the advice about learning to say "No". And begin your new, slim life — as a Water sign, you do like to get things moving!

LEO

July 23 — August 22

Ruled by the Sun, the centre of our solar system and the prime source of light and heat, Leos are motivated by a burning desire to initiate action. The constellation of Leo is very noticeable in the night sky. It is bright, easy to spot - a strong indication that people born under this sign stand out in a crowd and possess the ability to gain attention easily. Leo, which is the fifth sign of the zodiac, is symbolised by the Lion, the powerful king of the jungle. Associated with the element of Fire, this is a sign that governs one of the hottest astrological months in the northern hemisphere.

<u>YOUR SLIMMING CHARACTER</u>

The state of your figure often reflects your current ambitions. You throw yourself wholeheartedly into any cause which fires your imagination and that is the time when you're less inclined to depend on edible props to get you through each day. As a Leo it is especially easy for you to be noticed and remembered. But although you know how to steal the limelight, at times you also need to disappear quietly into the background — and this is when you may have a snack too many. A pity, because when you do make an appearance, it is important for your self-esteem to know that you look good and that your figure is able to stand up to close scrutiny.

The Sun is the ruler of your sign, and like the sun you have an inner need to shine and be appreciated. Your need for approval is a vital point to remember. The respect you will earn from your friends and family, by proving you have the will-power to slim down to the supple, lithe being that is really you — this well-earned respect will encourage you to make your new way of eating and drinking your norm.

As the "fixed" fire sign, you will use this slimming book with enthusiasm. Once you believe in anything, you rarely waiver or change your mind. The "fixed" quality of Leo gives you loyalty to a cause or a belief. You would not be reading this book if you had not already made up your mind that it holds exciting possibilities. Indeed, when you open this book there is no doubt you will be tucked away somewhere on your own, wishing to investigate it and try it out first, before you admit to anyone else that you have read it. It is usually all or nothing with you, and if you like what you read, not only will you be recommending this book to others, but it will probably be high on your list as a special gift for your friends and family members.

YOUR SLIMMING STRENGTHS

Pride in yourself and the way you look represents one of your greatest strengths so far as staying slim and healthy is concerned. The knowledge that you can dress up in smart, trendy clothes that make an impact, whenever you like, without feeling embarrassed about your shape, is the perfect incentive for you to lose weight as necessary. The reward of being able to show off your new, slim profile is well worth working for. Criticism is also a wonderful spur to you to improve your image. Although someone else's chance remark can dent your ego, it can act like a trigger to set you off on a determined fitness or slimming course.

TAKING YOUR MEDICINE
It goes without saying that you should consult your doctor before changing your diet if you have any kind of physical heart problem, but if you're suffering from a heart problem of the emotional sort, it may pay you to consult your best friend rather than trying to 'doctor' yourself with a comforting eclair or a large gin and tonic!

Even as a child, your parents and teachers must have had to handle you with respect because your strong will and ability to stick to your guns indicated a refusal to budge unless you wanted to. You cannot fail to succeed in your efforts to slim if you muster this willpower now and keep your ultimate goal clearly in sight. Your resolute nature and determination, as well as the diets in this book, will provide the winning formula to slim, so set yourself a realistic target weight today.

Another of your qualities, your self-discipline, is a great slimming strength , and just what's required for you to stick to a steady and effective routine. Never doubt that you can achieve the weight loss you seek, because the stubborn side of your personality is unlikely to give up once you start. Even in one week you will begin to see and feel the benefits.

When you put your mind to it, you are unsurpassed in the art of persuasion, so should have no difficulty in coaxing your family and friends to support your efforts to look after what is one of your greatest assets — your body.

You tend to dress up or down, according to the shape of your figure, so it is obvious that you must stay in control of your weight once you have regained your desired size. As you begin to follow your diet programme, remember you have taken an important and very positive step towards doing something for yourself. By all means enlist the support and encouragement of your friends and other members of your household, but don't worry if you have to go it alone, because you have reserves of courage which you should now recognise, and are usually prepared to hold your ground when facing opposition. The company of other people is good for Leo morale, but bear in mind that it is down to you to set the pace.

You hate people to feel sorry for you, because it is easier for you to be the giver rather than the receiver of sympathy. Remember this, especially if you intend to diet along with a Leo friend who is overweight. Let them believe that they are helping you to stick to your diet, rather than the other way around.

Leos, both men and women, are good organisers and leaders of others — so turn this organising flair to your advantage by planning a healthy diet for the whole family, "adjusting" the size of the portions accordingly. You have high ideals and the power to inspire others to work for you — and with you. But all your leadership and drive can be wasted unless you establish a direction and have a clear-cut plan. Make your plan one that is beneficial to your health and one that will also boost your confidence.

You possess a certain dignity and usually appear very self-

COVER-UPS
When buying new clothes, be firm with yourself and resist buying loose garments that camouflage your flab. Instead shop for the style you would really like to wear, even if you are bulging at the seams for the first few weeks of your diet. That Leo pride will act like a spur to your efforts to lose weight and soon have you streamlined all over.

assured, which makes you a natural manager, teacher and director of operations. You must now take even more control of your life-style, even if that means a total restructure of your shopping and eating habits. The part of you that quite likes to show off will be delighted when you can boast of your slimming achievements!

YOUR SLIMMING WEAKNESSES

Born in late July or August, you are ruled by the Sun, so rarely feel at your best when the weather is cold or depressing. The wintertime represents one of the most dangerous periods for your figure. Resist the tendency to turn to hot soup and stodgy but filling food for warmth and comfort if the temperature has dropped to below zero. Exercise is a far healthier way to warm up. But wrapping up against chilly winds and icy blasts will also stop your stomach from demanding food in order to put on a protective coating of insulating but unsightly fat, which unfortunately is likely to stay with you when the climate has become more amicable. Remember you can unzip an anorak more easily than you can unzip a layer of fat.

You tend to be a creature of habit; which is fine if your habits are healthy ones — those ones which you have consciously and wisely selected — but beware if they're not! Your habitual eating habits can be the direct cause of a progressive weight gain. Think back to when you were young and ask yourself whether you have allowed yourself to become accustomed to a style of eating which suited your heftier ancestors, but is gradually filling you out so that you are beginning to resemble the more generously endowed members of your family. Keep a note of every single morsel you normally consume; you would probably be surprised at just how often you eat or drink without being genuinely hungry or thirsty.

There is a generosity of spirit that is particular to Leos. This

HIDDEN FATTENERS

As a Leo, you like to eat in style, so be extra cautious about those apparently inoffensive nibbles that many restaurants serve while you're waiting. Salty snacks in particular make you want to keep on eating and drink more at the same time. Also ask how meat or fish has been cooked and opt for grilled rather than fried every time. Rich sauces and oily dressings are also bad news.

expansive, big-hearted characteristic can be another slimming obstacle. When you entertain, you do so grandly and in style. Only the best is good enough for your family and friends — you like quality as well as quantity. You must be especially careful when you are celebrating or enjoying a special meal, as the happy mood of the moment could prove to be an unfortunate one later if it causes an unwanted weight gain. Treat your body with as much care and consideration as you do your friends — after all you'll be together for a long time. Pretend you are entertaining one of your most valued friends and they are on a diet. Your natural desire to impress others means you gain most by trying to impress yourself.

The "fixed" quality of Leo can give you an element of stubbornness, which can make you resistant to change, even when it's good for you. Don't dig your heels in now, because there's only one way to attain that figure you've set your heart on and that is by changing your eating habits — in fact this could be the best change you've ever made.

Gold, which is Leo's metal, is used in the making of crowns — a sign of Leo's rulership qualities. Only the best is good enough for you. No one knows as well as you do that

> **WHAT'S YOURS?**
> *If you like a drink, be crafty and learn a few clever slimming dodges. Make yours a Spritzer — a mixture of white wine and soda water — highly fashionable and half the calories of a straight glass of wine. Low calorie mixers should be the rule if you drink spirits. Also favour low calorie lemonade or cola whenever you order, and always use a small glass rather than a large one. Bottled mineral water is a fun tipple which isn't fattening.*

you were born for great things. This taste for the high-life can make you want the lion's share of the cake, another obstacle to overcome where slimming is concerned.

YOU AND YOUR BODY

The heart and spine are the parts of the body particularly associated with Leo and problems of the heart, whether physical or emotional, invariably cause your weight to go haywire. Similarly, damage to your back or carrying too heavy an emotional load in the way of problems also have an adverse effect on your figure. Nevertheless, there's no doubt that you have the capacity to put your whole heart into everything you do. You are proud of the way you look and do not resent spending any money and time on keeping yourself in tip-top condition.

Your body is really your pride and joy and the better it looks, the better you feel, so to be always in peak condition is especially important to you.

You respond positively to the sun's warm rays which revitalise you and put you on top of the world, so gaining a sun tan can provide a great boost to your health as well as your morale. Just be sure to use a safe sunscreening cream.

Weigh in and measure your vital statistics at the same time each week — your waist, bust (or chest) and your hips and record them in your own slimming diary.

There's nothing like being presented with firm evidence of the true state of your figure to motivate you to slim down to the shape you once were, or have always wanted to be. Set diets suit you best and — because you like a challenge — you can aim for and achieve spectacular results in record time.

Gymnastics and cat-like exercises, which stretch your body and keep you lithe and supple, are ideal for you. Plan to walk tall and try to be aware of the way you move. Swimming and dancing provide you with the chance to tone up your muscles and relax at the same time, so these are also good for you.

Your fixed, fiery Leo temperament can cope with a rigid routine if you are given the right incentive. Leos can become keep-fit fanatics when they think that their natural good shape is at risk. This means that when you decide to diet, you stand every chance of achieving your goals in record time. Indeed, once you've made up your mind to take positive action, where your body's concerned, there's no stopping you.

SAFE SHOPPING

There's no doubt that Leos love to shop. But watch your shopping routine on Danger Days. At the supermarket, take a basket rather than a trolley — that way, you'll carry less home. If you can, leave your cheque book and credit cards at home and carry only the cash you've budgeted to spend. Female Leos can, best of all, take themselves to a department store with plenty of beauty counters. A new lipstick or bath lotion will perk up your morale. And if you must take a rest in the coffee shop or wine bar — order a mineral water.

YOU AND YOUR EMOTIONS

A loved Leo is a radiant Leo, one who has the ability to spread warmth, joy and sunshine all around. You are able to brighten up the world for others, and this wonderful gift is at a peak when you are in a good emotional relationship. As Leo is a Fire sign, you also possess a fiery spark within you — a spark that can light the way for others.

You prefer to lead rather than follow and like to choose your friends and partners, so usually make the first approach. Although you need time to be on your own, you also like to attract attention and affection. You usually make quite an impression on newcomers — a Leo rarely goes unnoticed. It is up to you whether you are remembered for your slim and healthy looks, or for your overweight shape.

Your partner's appearance is as important to you as your own, so if they are overweight you will soon tell them to do something about it — you can now set a good example by checking your Astrochart for your first suitable slimming date and getting started.

Being without a partner is especially hard for you to bear because you come into your own and do your best work when you have someone to do it for. And as much as you hate criticism, asking your opposite number or your best friend for an honest appraisal of your figure could be just the motivation you need to keep you on the straight and narrow when it comes to eating. Your desire to please and impress those you love is a wonderful slimming aid.

Your own ability to be consistent in your affections can lead you to expect the same behaviour from others, so you find it hard to accept if anyone lets you down. Keeping up a brave front is very important to you, so you don't always show it when you feel rebuffed or rejected. This reluctance to pour your heart out and find a shoulder to cry on, even when you have every reason to do so, can be counter-productive for your figure because suppressing hurt feelings is always risky for your diet intentions. Even so, you must guard against a tendency to dwell on and magnify problems. When you console yourself with food, you tend to do so in a grand manner, regardless of the consequences for your waistline!

You are passionate, loyal and a person of commitment. You instinctively respect the depth of feeling that the Water people possess, but are also aware that they can dampen your fiery enthusiasm — that is unless you make them feel good about what you're doing.

You expect to rule and make no bones about it. It is worth remembering that although those born under the Water signs — Cancers, Scorpios and Pisces — may seem submissive, the opposite is usually the case, so you could experience power struggles, albeit subtle ones, between yourself and Water people: they are masters of manipulation because they, too, want to control and often manage to do so without it becoming obvious. To share a diet plan with a Water person, be prepared to be nagged if you lapse, because little escapes their notice.

You'll have fun with another Fire person in the family. With a Leo like yourself, or an Aries or Sagittarius, you will spark each other, so could cause quite a stir. Any close relationship with a Fire person should be a lively and eventful one. As you share the desire for action with other Fire signs, they make wonderful diet companions for you.

Even so, you're ideally suited in a relationship with an Air person, who will both infuriate you with their curiosity and insistence on discussing the whys and wherefores of everything and fascinate you with their free thinking minds and wealth of ideas. Life with a Gemini, Libra or Aquarius is likely to be interesting and adventurous, as they will help you to broaden your outlook, examine yourself and your eating patterns objectively and encourage you to expand your horizons. Their laid-back attitudes to life will stop you exaggerating your slimming problems and help you to see how easy it is to follow your diet and find your perfect figure.

Earth sign people have qualities you admire — staying-power and practical, common sense. Many Leos team up with them, both on an emotional level and also in business. Your ability to be definite, positive and not wishy-washy goes down well with the less flamboyant signs of Taurus, Virgo and Capricorn. Announcing your intention to slim and shape up is enough to gain the support of your Earth partner or friends, because you reinforce their belief in themselves with your air of confidence — which you have even when you are feeling more like a pussy-cat than a lion!

YOUR CREATIVE ENERGIES

Yours is one of the most creative signs of the zodiac and it is by developing your potential talents that you gain self-respect and can take true pride in yourself and your accomplishments. Your spare-time activities often provide you with the creative outlets your work life sometimes lacks. You possess a most powerful energy to express yourself, so can quickly set plans into action and organise events. This power allows you to succeed in whatever area you are drawn to. You are an individualist, with a strong sense of drama. This is why many actors and entertainers are born when the Sun is in Leo. You come into your own when you are free to pursue your leisure activities. These should allow you to let your hair down and express your sunny personality. You need amusements which lighten your spirit. Laughing and making other people laugh represent great slimming boosts because having an optimistic and exuberant mood reinforces your sense of well-being — and counters any tendency to make friends with a comforting drink or a plate of French fries.

> **BEST FRIEND TACTIC**
> *Leos possess the gift of being able to bring the warmth of their Sun sign into the lives of others. But your urge to entertain with food and drink can be your slimming downfall. Next time you want to cheer up a sad Cancerian or a broken-hearted Pisces, remember that a long, cheery phone call costs nothing in calories.*

Making music, amateur dramatics, playing games, painting, sketching are all Leo pursuits, but preferably with an appreciative audience to commend your efforts. Involving yourself in activities which are pleasing to you will help you to diet because you will be concentrating on pouring out your energies instead of taking in additional energy in the form of food.

Spur of the moment entertaining is not really your style because you like to plan ahead and usually put careful thought into every detail, from the menu to the way the table is laid. Presentation is all-important to you, so to avoid missing out on the sauces and toppings you like, learn to substitute a low-calorie variety.

Being able to relax completely is an essential part of a holiday for you, and even when you go on an activity holiday you tend to allow for a couple of days to do absolutely nothing, lazing in the sun, preferably on a sandy beach in some exotic part of the world. Invest in some sunshine whenever you can — it bucks up your spirits and reinforces your will-power: aim to make that body of yours a perfect picture, so you'll be proud when you hand round your holiday snaps.

VIRGO

August 23 — September 22

Although the Greek word 'zodiac' means the circle of animals, Virgo is symbolised by the Virgin, depicted as a young girl, indicating the untapped resources in Man. And it is by recognising and using their talents to their full potential, that Virgos become fulfilled. Virgo is one of the three mutable (or adaptable) signs, giving Virgos versatility and also a certain restless quality. However, as Virgo is a one of the stable Earth signs, they also seek security. Virgo is the sign of service and those born under this sign possess an urge to be of value to others, so are often happy in a supporting role. The planetary ruler of Virgo is Mercury, the planet of communication.

YOUR SLIMMING CHARACTER

Being a Virgo can be exhausting. Similar to a computer, you analyse, sift and store every single scrap of information presented to you. Your ability to observe and not miss the tiniest detail makes you a model slimming candidate, as you will be meticulous about following your diet plan.

Virgos are perhaps the most health-conscious of all the zodiac signs: you have a natural interest in your body and what fuels it. You may already be clued up on calories and food values. You will, therefore, warmly appreciate the winning format of a diet which has taken these into account. Your diet also caters for a liking for order, which you share with the other Earth signs, Taurus and Capricorn. You also share your ruling planet, Mercury, with the Air sign of Gemini and, like a Gemini, tend to be restless, wanting to be constantly on the move. Unfortunately, no matter how much you move around, you stand as much chance of becoming overweight as any of the other eleven signs! That is why you will benefit from following a structured plan of eating, one which provides you with plenty of energy to meet the demands of your busy, bustling life.

YOUR SLIMMING WEAKNESSES

Those born under your sign are considered to be especially adaptable and flexible, which can be a problem where slimming's concerned. Your readiness to alter your arrangements at the drop of a hat can result in irregular eating patterns and erratic weight gains and losses, instead of the steady reduction that represents sensible slimming — vital if you are to achieve your desired weight in the best of health and retain it on the long term.

You are fully aware of the importance of eating sufficient food and not missing too many meals, because you know that no-one, not even you, can be effective and function well if they are deprived of nourishment for long periods. But ask yourself, do you sometimes exist all day on a few cups of black coffee and an apple, only to sit down to a mammoth meal in the evening and then waddle your way to bed? Eating sensible portions of food at regular intervals is essential if you are to slim down your surplus flab — and stay slim. Resolve to avoid stocking up your fuel tanks in one fell swoop, especially late in the day. Eating immediately before bed-time is not the way to burn up your fat. A brisk walk after a meal tones up your circulation and allows your body to convert your food to energy.

WANDERING HANDS

You need spare time activities that occupy your hands as well as your thoughts, or you soon become very fidgety. The next time you feel tempted to ferret in a bag of nuts or unwrap a packet of biscuits, remember: it's not your stomach but your hands that need to be gainfully employed.

At the same time, another Virgo practice to be severely discouraged is eating an extra helping of pie or potatoes in case you have no time to grab a snack later. Not only does this expand your stomach, which then wants more, and more, but you also create an unwanted store-cupboard of plump fat cells.

One of your greatest slimming weaknesses is your reluctance to see good food go to waste. This can lead you to finishing up the leftovers to save them being thrown out if they're not eaten. You're particularly at risk if you're raising a young family, as many a young Virgo parent has started a premature middle-aged spread by helping junior out with his or her dinner. It may help you if someone else could serve your meals and be responsible for removing any tempting tit-bits which remain on the table at the end of a meal.

You like to be well-informed, and have an uncanny knack for assimilating all sorts of facts and figures — no doubt you know more about 'E' numbers, the effects of food colourings and the need your brain has for the essential 'B' vitamins, than most of your friends. Nevertheless, even you can fail to appreciate the hidden calories in many of your favourite health foods, especially in pulses, nuts and brown bread. Remember, the size of a portion of food is an unreliable guide to its fattening potential — your Astrodiet will work because it allows you to have bulk without bulges and also eat healthily and enjoy your meals at the same time.

Even if you're not a dedicated party-goer or socialite, you usually have the gift of bringing people together when there's a purpose, so you find yourself the organiser of many events. Your friends and associates are likely to view you as a useful person to know. This means that many invitations to wine, dine and make merry do seem to come your way as you go through life. Another obstacle to sticking to a slimming diet. Your Astrochart gives the dates when your will-power could be weaker than usual, so try to avoid attending social functions at these times, if given a choice.

Keep a diary and enter your "danger days", so you can plan accordingly when taking bookings. In your personal life and your employment, you must try to guard against pressures building up. If for financial, family, or emotional reasons you are unable to organise your affairs in the smooth-running way you prefer, you sometimes take your frustration out on your figure by eating extra to requirements. Remember, your slimming campaign is one area of your life which can follow a predictable pattern and cause no anxiety or aggravations because your diet has been designed with your personality in mind.

NO TO TEMPTATION
Avoid creating your own temptation, as from today, by making an immediate resolution never to set one foot inside a supermarket or your local corner shop without a list. As a painstaking Virgo, this shouldn't be hard to organise. And close your eyes firmly to 'special offers' of the fattening variety — remember a lower price today could mean a higher weight tomorrow!

YOUR SLIMMING STRENGTHS

You are a perfectionist with the ability to be your own slave-driver when it comes to correcting any imperfections in the way you look. This is one of your greatest slimming strengths. Losing weight cannot alter your basic body type, the one you have inherited from your ancestors, but by ridding yourself of surplus fat, you can achieve the perfect weight, the one that is right for your height and good for your health.

Another of your strengths is the way you break down large, formidable projects into smaller, more manageable tasks. This helps you to achieve the seemingly impossible, so if you want to change your life, start here — with your weight. And remember that one change invariably leads to another. The love, the job, the social life you seek, become one step closer when you know that you radiate confidence — the confidence that comes from feeling healthy and looking dynamic, especially as you know that you are ready to slog away long after others would have given up. Definitely a plus factor for your slimming aspirations.

> **START THINKING THIN**
> *The Virgo's mind is usually buzzing about one thing or another. But at times you expect too much of yourself. Set a monthly slimming target and be satisfied when you reach it.*

There is a thrifty side to your nature which demands value for money. You are sensible enough to live within your means, so put a lot of thought into how you spend your cash. You're not fooled by fancy trimmings and expensive labels, you are a realist, who doesn't judge a book by its cover. You will appreciate the economic sense of only shopping for, and eating, what is needed, rather than buying impulsively in your local delicatessen or supermarket; especially when you see your bank balance grow larger, instead of your waistline.

Virgo, as already mentioned, is one of the most adaptable signs of the zodiac. Your ability to change your ways and your habits to suit the changing demands of your environment, equip you well for following this diet.

Fortunately, like all Earth signs, you can recognise a promising format when you see one. Make sure you consult your Astrochart before you begin your slimming regime however, because that security-conscious side to your nature needs to know that your chances of success are at a high. As you are shrewd enough to recognise useful hints, whether they are given intentionally or not, it will also pay you to swap slimming stories with your colleagues, neighbours and friends.

You are a careful person but not over-cautious. You also have staying power, as well as the curiosity, to give this new way of dieting the chance it deserves by following each week through conscientiously, until it becomes obvious, as it soon will, that your Astrodiet really works. Although you may dismiss your initial weight loss as a lucky coincidence (because you are not easily impressed) you will be delighted with the fact that once you have slimmed down you can retain your target weight with minimum hassle.

Although, as has already been pointed out, there can be certain drawbacks in your liking for healthy foods, due to the high calorific rate of many products found in a health store, there are also advantages. The interest you have in the working of your body means that you instantly recognise, and are also honest with yourself, when the food

HI-TECH SLIMMING

As a Virgo, you appreciate good food, so why not treat yourself to a few gadgets which will make the food preparation as much fun as eating it? New shredders, blenders, graters and slicers will also give your mind plenty of food for thought and help you enjoy your slimming days even more.

and drink you consume is not really good for you. Just think how good you'll feel when you know that every bite you take is exactly what your body needs and a step towards becoming slimmer and more energetic!

YOU AND YOUR BODY

Your natural interest in body matters is sometimes misunderstood, so may have earned you the undeserved title of being a hypochondriac. In reality, you are usually a fairly healthy sign, with a good chance of living to a ripe old age. Like the other two Earth signs, Taurus and Capricorn, you possess staying-power, so will be able to stick with your diet.

Like Mercury, your ruling planet, it's natural for you to be energetic which means you are at your healthiest and happiest when you have plenty to keep you occupied. But even though yours is a very active sign, you do tend to put on weight as you grow older — that is unless you are one of those lucky petite, small-boned Virgos, who stay slim all their lives, no matter how much they eat. But if this is the case, you're more likely to be reading this book out of curiosity than for any other reason!

It is essential for you to learn to relax and accept life as it comes, instead of constantly analysing every potential problem, as well as those that actually exist. Do you find that you leave your home half an hour before you need to, in case you are late? And phone your friends twice in order to double-check your arrangements, sometimes infuriating them in the process? This Virgo trait of inspecting every minute detail in a plan to make sure that nothing goes wrong, is bound to take its toll on your nervous system. You can waste a lot of time and effort unless you learn the power of positive thought, because your nerves, abdomen and intestines are the parts of the body particularly associated with Virgo, and these can act like a barometer to the pressures which build up. Your high standards of perfection can make you worry more than most if your body's size, shape or physical condition is not as it should be, so having a fit, healthy and slim body will raise your morale as well as your vitality.

LOW COST FLAVOUR

Here's another tip which is sure to appeal to the thrifty side of your Virgo nature. Using a microwave oven takes so little fuel that you are actually saving on your bills. Apart from the economical good sense, you will win by cutting down on those unsavoury smells which waft through your home when you're cooking fish or vegetables — and they taste far better.

Sticking to your diet will also be a wonderful aid to your digestion. Like your opposite sign, Pisces, you may display extremist behaviour when it comes to your eating habits. You can alternate between half-starving yourself one minute, because you are too busy to prepare yourself a meal, and over-indulging yourself the next. The portions suggested in your Astrodiet plan will remove any uncertainty you have about how much, or how little, to eat.

In fact moderation in all things is a sound policy for you to adopt. You should aim for a gradual weight loss and take regular exercise — remember there's no need to be an athlete to exercise your body. In any case aggressive sports and work-outs are not really your style. Generally your exercise plan should lean towards straightforward, repetitive techniques.

Go for the kind of exercise that you can do every day, and may do already in your everyday life, such as walking or cycling. These will assist your weight reduction campaign, and also help to prevent many of the usual age-related health problems associated with bone and muscle degeneration.

YOU AND YOUR EMOTIONS

On the outside you are cool, calm and unruffled; on the inside you are warm, earthy and sensual. Having a partner is important to your sense of security. It is easy for you to make friends because your pleasant manner does not intimidate others. Mercury rules your sign, so you are rarely at a loss for words and can strike up a conversation with most people, while at the same time you are an attentive listener. If you like what you see, you can go to a great deal of trouble to cultivate a partnership, but you usually think very carefully before giving your heart. Once you fall in love, you are a person of devotion and will do your utmost to sustain your relationship. This commitment and dedication to a person, or a cause, can now be applied successfully in your campaign to lose weight.

It is in your very nature to try to please others, to back them up, prop them up and protect them from hardship. One of your life's lessons is to learn to discriminate between when help is wanted and when it isn't, because at times your involvement in other people's problems can be unwanted. To be happy in love, it is important that you feel needed, so you need a partner who is not too independent or ungrateful. At times, you can sacrifice your own interests and priorities in order to meet a loved-one's demands. You should now concentrate on pleasing yourself. The right to be slim and more attractive is not only for others. And later, when you have shed your unwanted fat, you may find you can be of service to an overweight member of your circle by showing them that they, too, can "Slim by the Stars."

Casual romance is not your style because you seek permanency and loyalty from a partner. You are usually extremely tolerant of other people's quirks and failings. Fortunately, as you tend to be a good judge of character, you are not easily taken by surprise. You need someone who will value the many little things you do to make them happy. It's in your nature to fetch, carry and fuss over the object of your affections. Ideally, they should also stimulate you mentally and share your distinctive brand of humour.

Another Virgo, or someone born under one of the other Earth

signs, will appreciate your supportive attitudes and share your liking for a settled existence. This can be a good combination for a life-long relationship with few disagreements, but could lack the spontaneity and sense of adventure that can add a sparkle to life. Slimming with an Earth partner should go like clockwork, as you both accept discipline and rules, especially if you have set your sights on a weight-loss goal.

Teaming up with one of the Air people, Gemini, Libra or Aquarius brings many conflicting aspects into play. They deal in abstracts and theories, while you prefer realities and facts. You can benefit from each other's different approach, whether sharing a home, or your fight against the flab. You can help them regulate their eating patterns and they can help you forget your worries and give you a thousand and one reasons to press on with your diet.

You will feel at home with a Water person, a Cancer, Scorpio or Pisces, as they will respond instinctively to you and appreciate your caring qualities. All Water people seek a permanent anchor for their strong emotions, so will welcome you with open arms, while you will derive great pleasure from feeling indispensable. As a slimming team, you will soon find success because the mutual understanding and sympathy between you will ensure that neither of you buy temptation or place it on the dinner table.

Fire people and you are poles apart. They are urgent, impatient and eager for action, whereas you are cautious, patient and restrained. As opposites tend to attract, Fire people will excite you with their energy and colour and they will be drawn to your quiet strength and composure. Slimming with a Fire partner could be infuriating at times. Only eat your meals with them if they are trying to slim too, or you will be constantly defending your decisions not to put butter on your vegetables or serve the fish without a pile of chips.

YOUR CREATIVE ENERGIES

If you are a typical Virgo, you tend to evaluate your days on how much you have achieved, so need to find the kind of outlet for your creative energies which will produce tangible results. You usually gain more satisfaction from looking at the lawn you have carefully laid or the sweater you knitted, than from a session of hang gliding or from walking aimlessly. There has to be a sensible reason for whatever you do, so no doubt you appreciate all of the reasons behind staying slim.

Your taste in books veers towards fact, rather than fiction.

Autobiographies, real life dramas, natural history, art, politics are all popular Virgo reading. Your personal collection of books probably rivals the local library, as collecting is a Virgo hobby. Miniature portraits, interesting glass bottles, unusual handicrafts, old gramophone records and brass rubbings are typical Virgo passions. One thing you cannot afford to collect, however, is fat, because it will reduce your mobility and can undermine your confidence.

SIPPING STRATEGY
Your diet calls for you to drink 6 - 8 glasses of water a day. (Designer water if you prefer.) Progamme this into your daily lifestyle. If you can, take the chance to sit down for a while. Then as you sip, write down a plan for the clothes you'll buy, or the holiday you'll take, once you've achieved your slimming goal.

Your way of unwinding is to immerse yourself in your hobbies, but you tend to do more than one thing at a time. Do you find that you write a letter and watch television at the same time, or hold an in-depth telephone conversation whilst whipping up an omelette?

Like most Virgos, you may like to travel and explore the world, scrimping and saving if necessary to be able to take off to distant parts or pastures new. Organized tours with running commentaries were designed for a Virgo, who hates to miss a thing. You probably swot up on places of interest, the local history, customs and even the language of any place that you visit. You cast your critical eye over the foreign vino and cuisine, taste it and pass your judgement. If you like it, it had better be low in calories, or you will return from your journey fatter as well as fitter.

You are a good mixer, but are inclined to divide your time between meeting your friends and spending time alone. You are not really a pace-setter, but often take responsibility in groups, for example on a committee, because you are conscientious and can also be relied upon to spot what others have missed. This exacting side of your personality helps you to succeed in home crafts and D.I.Y. projects, because you leave nothing to chance. This perfectionist quality is also the reason you can be certain of achieving your target weight by following your Astrodiet.

LIBRA

September 23 — October 22

The Sun enters Libra, the sign of balance, at one of the two times of the year when the hours of daylight equal the hours of darkness (the other is in March when the Sun enters Aries) and all Librans place great store on retaining a balance in their lives. Libra's planetary ruler Venus is the third brightest celestial body after the Sun and Moon. Venus is a planet associated with love and harmony and Librans are rarely happy without both of these. Libra is the seventh sign of the zodiac and the cardinal (or leading) Air sign. In common with the other Air signs Gemini and Aquarius, it is vital for all Librans to be allowed enough space and freedom to follow their own interests.

YOUR SLIMMING CHARACTER

Sometimes the Libran scales say "Ouch!" because balancing your weight and your lifestyle can be one of the most difficult juggling tricks of all for you. A balanced routine and a harmonious lifestyle are essential to you if you are to maintain a steady weight, one which doesn't swing from one extreme to another according to what's happening in your life.

Your ruling planet Venus was considered by the ancient astrologers to be a sign of love and good luck as well as of beauty and harmony. It is, therefore, especially important for you to have a body that pleases your eye. Wanting to be slim and attractive is not necessarily vanity in your case, but a genuine feeling of distress when you know that you are not looking your best. A good enough reason for you to start your slimming diet on the next suitable date given in your Astrochart.

If you're a typical Libran, you yearn for a world which is stress-free and without pain. In fact, it is the lack of peace and tranquillity in your life that is often an underlying cause of your overweight problems, because it upsets your equilibrium. It is by creating harmony and a beautiful world for yourself that you can become fulfilled and stay healthy and slim.

YOUR SLIMMING WEAKNESSES

The most difficult part of starting a new project for you is initiating the action. No-one is more expert than you at putting things off, so you are often labelled the "ditherer of the zodiac". All too often you wait for a decision to be forced upon you before you direct your energies into a new scheme or make a change. Although your intentions may be sincere, the motivation to make a start is sometimes lacking. Your Astrochart will remove the uncertainty about whether or not the time is right for you to begin your new diet plan. You rarely act on impulse as you prefer to weigh up the advantages and disadvantages before making a commitment of any kind.

For you, life is about constantly striving towards finding harmony — both harmony of your head and your heart, and harmony between yourself and other people. You want to be friends with everyone, and hate to say "No", which is one of your slimming obstacles because a cross word, or a steely silence can send you scuttling to the biscuit tin or the drinks cupboard.

TREAT YOURSELF

Food is often a prime source of comfort to you, so make sure that what you eat looks good, spending time over preparation and present-ation - there's no need for diet dishes to be dull. Whether you eat from a tray or at a table, make it look inviting and if you know that you're inclined to nibble when you're upset, consider non-edible forms of consolation, such as a bunch of flowers or a good book.

Your Astrochart will help you to know in advance when you must take evasive action, so that you do not give anyone who has the power to upset you, the power to upset your diet plan.

Another area of vulnerability for you is your Libran tendency to give and receive presents, so as an aspiring Libran sylph, ask your friends and family for gifts of the non-edible variety, as unwrapping a birthday present which is begging to be eaten, can be disastrous so far as your weight is concerned. You are also at risk when you are bored, with little to do, or immobile because you're watching television or reading a book, as both of these situations tempt you to nibble.

You are usually a good mixer because you are tactful and unassuming. When entertaining, you possess the knack of taking care of all the little touches which make your guests feel comfortable and relaxed. The food and arrangements will be presented with care and great thought. BUT you must put as much thought into what you eat, especially at a social get-together. As Venus, planet of comfortable living, rules your sign, the chances are that even your first tooth was a sweet one.

Also, be ruthless with leftovers when you entertain others. Why not provide your guests with a "doggie bag" and put the onus on them whether or not to eat up any surplus gateau or party fare?

Another slimming weakness you must watch for, is a tendency to bury your head in the sand if there is a problem you don't want to face. Where the battle of overweight is concerned, your problem is unlikely to go away. You cannot escape the harsh fact that it's up to you to put matters right. If you follow your diet plan on a regular basis you will eventually sort out your problems.

As you will note in your Astrochart, there will be Danger days when it will take twice as much determination to stay with your diet. These days are more threatening to you than they are to the less sensitive signs, because if you encounter a set-back by exceeding your permitted intake of food, it could undermine your confidence. Regard any such set-back, if one should occur, as only a temporary lapse, write it off to experience and continue with your diet plan as if nothing had happened.

YOUR SLIMMING STRENGTHS

As a Libran, you're potentially an ideal candidate for a structured slimming plan (as offered in this book) because you respond well to the idea of a balanced diet, created with your personality in mind. You can confidently indulge your love of socialising on your "good" days in your Astrochart, when Venus is ensuring that you will be full of the joys of life and, therefore, able to enjoy food without over-indulging. As you tend to be less strong-willed when Venus is at odds with Libra, you should keep a constant check on your Astrocharts, so that you can stay out of temptation's way during

AIM TO PLEASE
You like to please, so treat your body in the way you treat your best friend — considerately, with love and attention. But instead of treating yourself to a box of chocolates on your birthday, splash out on perfumed bath fragrances or a luxury body oil. After all, the slimmer you become the longer it will last.

your Ddanger days. You will go to great lengths to look good if there is someone you wish to impress. This is one of your greatest slimming strengths, so use it to your advantage. Make a regular habit of meeting up with people who motivate you to dress up and look your best. The more often you arrange to get together with those you wish to attract, the better, as you'll work hard to present a dynamic image. You also benefit from meeting people who tend to look you up and down and judge you by your appearance, as knowing you'll be under the spotlight spurs you on to achieve your target weight. You'll want to be slim, even if they are bulging at the seams. Socialise whenever possible: catching up on old school chums is always a winner, as you would be ashamed to let them see you a few sizes larger than when you graduated. You cannot cope with harsh criticism, especially when you know there is something you could do about your size and shape. In fact, the more severe the appraisal you receive, the more incentive you have to stick to your slimming plan.

GRILL THRILL
Grilling grapefruit adds no calories — try it this way as a breakfast or main meal starter. If you consider cottage cheese to be a trifle boring, use it as the basis for a mixed salad. Chop, grate or slice salad vegetables, and stir into the cheese. On the days when you are allowed bread, cubed dry toast makes a scrunchy extra.

In your personal book of rules you believe that endeavour should be rewarded Equally, you don't expect to enjoy results without making an effort. The Libran symbol, the pair of delicately balanced scales, reflects the sensitivity you feel towards justice and fair play. The expectation you have that you will reap what you sow is another of your strengths in regard to slimming as you are prepared to stick to a discipline as long as you can see a continuous weight loss. You above all people know that everything has its price. Your scrupulous sense of justice will be worth its weight in gold in your daily diet plan, as you can be ruthlessly honest with yourself. You will be the first to admit it, if you break your diet in any way. All you need to do, as a way of atonement, is to sentence yourself to an extra day of dieting for the one you gave up on, and examine the reasons behind your lapse, so that you can take preventative measures in the future.

If you are true to your sign, you possess a natural charm, which makes others feel at ease in your company. No doubt you find that even comparative strangers confide in you. This isn't surprising because you are a wonderful listener. This is definitely a plus factor for dieting. Once you have heard other people's slimming-failure stories you will be all the keener to show that you can succeed.

Another important motivation for you to attain your desired shape is the inner knowledge that beauty is yours by birthright. To be slim and feel attractive is important to your sense of worth. Constantly visualise yourself as the shapely person you know you are inwardly, wearing the clothes that you would like to wear. If you stick to your diet, you will soon be wearing them.

YOU AND YOUR BODY

The theme of balance extends to your health habits as well as your material and emotional worlds. To stay slim, fit and energetic, you must balance inactive periods with time for exercise and without too much or too little of either. If you sit all day at a desk, organise action-packed sessions in the evening or at the weekends. Squash and other aggressive physical sports may be just what you need if you're deprived of physical outlets in your daily occupation. Conversely, if you're a busy housewife, or spend most of the day on your feet, rushing around, opt for gentle and calming pastimes which help you to relax and unwind. Meditation is ideal.

Also, weigh up your current eating habits with those you had as a child and identify which of your food likes and dislikes are hangovers from your early years and no longer in keeping with your body's requirements.

FRUIT TO SUIT
Eat your daily fruit allowance to suit yourself — between meals or as a starter or dessert. In fact, there doesn't have to be any set order in the way you eat. You can spread out your daily food allowance to make as many, or as few, meals as you want. Just help yourself from something on your daily list, whenever you feel like indulging in the odd snack, or treating yourself to a little something with your elevenses.

As a Libran, your body is particularly sensitive to the wear and tear of everyday life. Subjecting yourself to too much pressure or emotional disturbance soon makes its mark on your physical being. Headaches, backaches, stomach aches and generally feeling out of sorts are usually the direct result of a conflict or an unsatisfactory situation in your work, family or love life. You are more able to stay slim and healthy when your life is ticking over quietly, than when you are involved in heavy dramas or going through periods of stress or uncertainty.

Yours is an Air sign and it follows that fresh air is therapeutic to you. If you are to derive maximum benefit from an exercise plan, it must include opportunities to get out of doors. Don't despair if being cooped up has caused you to pile on the pounds and expanded your vital statistics — you can usually knock yourself into shape fairly rapidly once you're given the right motivation. Team up with a friend or your opposite number to join an exercise class or even a slimming club.

The parts of your body that are particularly associated with your sign are the lumbar region (the small of the back) and the kidneys.

YOU AND YOUR EMOTIONS

Conversation is an important part of your loving. The lack of someone to talk to, when you need company, can drive you to the fridge for other, less healthy types of distraction: such as puddings and chocolate bars, which only create another problem for you — that of being overweight. It is important that you find the courage to make the commitments called for in love, as not only do you have a great deal to offer the partner of your choice, but your bathroom scales quickly reflect the state of your emotions, by showing a gain in weight whenever you feel that you're missing out on love and affection, and a weight reduction when things are going well.

As already mentioned, the key qualities of your sign are

PICTURE THIS
Dig out your old photographs and have pictures of both the fattest and the slimmest members of your family in your kitchen. This will remind you in no uncertain terms of your options whenever you're preparing food. Don't fool yourself that you have inherited your extra inches, it's more likely that you were conditioned, as a child, to eat larger portions than your body needs.

balance and sharing, so it follows that you seek relationships that are based on mutual giving and taking. Feeling incomplete, either because you lack someone to share with, or because you are involved in an out-of-balance relationship — maybe a partnership in which you are doing most of the giving — can prove very disruptive for your eating habits.

You are rarely fulfilled on your own, but you cannot cope well with people who have overpowering or possessive personalities. Although, as a peace-lover, you are prepared to make allowances for those you love, you need to be realistic about what to expect from others, as of all the signs of the zodiac, yours is the one most likely to spend an entire life searching for your other half.— your soul mate who represents your perfect partner. That can be Libra's big mistake — to miss out on a love that is readily available just because the bearer comes complete with the usual share of human failings.

If your life partner is a fellow Libran, or born under one of the other Air signs, Gemini or Aquarius, your relationship could be the answer to your slimming prayers, because they will distract your thoughts from eating and be happy to spend time chatting to you whenever you feel a self-indulgent mood coming on. One thing you share with the other Air people is the ability to rationalise your own behaviour, so discussing your slimming strengths and weaknesses will help you understand yourself a little better. Your sense of humour and attitudes to life have many similarities — a good reason to find at least one Air person to compare notes with when slimming.

Aries, Leo and Sagittarius are signs associated with the element of Fire. The natural bounce, energy and directness of these people will both amuse and exasperate you. You can learn a lot from their willingness to take a chance, while they will profit from watching how you carefully analyse every situation and every probability before you take the plunge. You can expect some remarkable results if you diet with a Fire person, because you make a wonderful combination for success, especially as any excuse you make for lapsing in your diet will almost certainly be challenged.

You are often strongly attracted to the Water people, Cancer, Scorpio and Pisces, because their very difference appeals to you. Water people judge life by what they feel and by the impressions they receive, responding instinctively to the mood of the moment, while you plan your moves and consider what you are going to say, relying on your reasoning power to guide you.

Slimming with a Water person could open your eyes to many aspects of your eating patterns that you have failed to recognise, as they will sense immediately what effect your food is having on your body and will let you know in no uncertain terms if your diet is bad news.

A relationship with a Taurus, Virgo or Capricorn, the Earth signs, could prove extremely productive for you. Earth people are builders who like to have a structured plan to life. They are usually ready to work towards their goals and will also take a calculated risk as necessary. An Earth partner would offer you the steady support that your Airy personality needs and provide you with a strong shoulder to cry on in your times of troubles. At the same time, your gift of being able to look beyond the obvious will help them widen their horizons and they will also benefit from your questioning mind and flow of ideas. Even so, you could clash occasionally because Earth people seek containment, while you seek freedom. As all Earth people like to organise, they will appreciate the structure of your diet plan and help you to sort out your meal-time arrangements.

YOUR CREATIVE ENERGIES

Librans are well represented in the world of art and literature because yours is a creative sign. Painting, drawing, fashion, photography, collecting beautiful pictures and possessions, these are representative of your hobbies, or even your occupation. You often excel in other creative areas, such as writing and design, because you're an "ideas" person who is not unduly influenced by other people's suggestions and thoughts. Make a decision to involve yourself in interests which occupy your mind, whenever you feel inclined to eat out of boredom, as even if you prefer to observe rather than participate, all forms of dramatic display, such as the theatre, films and those activities which feature creative expression, stimulate you and please the imaginative side of your nature.

As freedom is so essential to your Airy sign, you should plan your holidays and your spare-time activities so you can visit the wide open spaces, as often as possible. Opt for packed lunches you have prepared for yourself from your daily allowance and avoid fattening but filling sausage-rolls or other savouries wrapped in pastry. Munch an apple or a carrot to allay any sudden pangs of hunger that tempt you to eat in between meals.

The sheer pleasure you derive from breathing in the pure, fresh air of the big outdoors revitalises you and helps you to cope with the demands of your everyday world. A contributing factor to successful dieting for you. Your need to escape from boring routine is one of the reasons you try to pack so much into your spare time. Don't hesitate to set the pace socially or to suggest the menus when eating out, because you have what it takes to play leader to others. You are equally happy when someone else takes charge, providing they discuss every detail with you first: this means you can have a say when it comes to the choice of refreshments and so be sure that the food you eat is not damaging to your diet.

Discussion and shared interest groups are right up your street, so it can be a good idea to join a slimming club or team up with fellow slimmers. Comparing notes will provide an extra boost to your intentions. Check out your Astrochart to discover the right day to make an approach in this matter.

SOME LIKE IT HOT
Hot up your main dishes with spices and herbs. You can add chilli to the mince and kidney beans, curry powder to the chicken, and so on. For an eye-catching salad remember that peppers come in many shades of red, green and yellow. If you like soup, use some of your vegetable allowance for it and try adding a shake or two of ginger powder to ring the changes.

Not only do you take your leisure moments extremely seriously, you usually have a built in clock which tells you when it's time for work to end and for play to begin, and vice-versa. It is when you ignore your own warning signs to ease up, or conversely to start moving, that your energy becomes depleted. Your spirits then begin to dampen and your thoughts turn to food. Balance and harmony — those words used so much in this chapter — are vital to your health and well-being: they are your personal formula for staying slim.

SCORPIO

October 23 — November 21

Scorpio, which is the eighth sign of the zodiac, is easy to spot in the heavens because it is the largest of the twelve constellations. Two Planets rule Scorpio: Mars, associated with energy and drive, and Pluto, planet of power and regeneration. Scorpio is the "fixed" (or stable) Water sign, suggesting that those born under this sign have hidden depths and are fluid in their thinking, but resistant to change. Like the Scorpion, the symbol of this sign, Scorpios are often fiercely self-protective with a strong survival instinct and a need for security.

YOUR SLIMMING CHARACTER

Birth, death and sex are associated with your sign, so you may have noticed a distinct pattern of beginnings and endings throughout your life, representing your personal "deaths" and "rebirths". Unlike some of the other signs, who are frequently given several options at the same time, it is rare for a new door to open for you before you've closed the previous one. The way for you to slim and feel completely reborn is to turn your back completely on your old way of eating — scrap those unsatisfactory eating habits once and for all, and start afresh. Your strong sense of self-preservation and desire to win, which make you a force to be reckoned with, can now be turned to your advantage — you can protect your own health and vitality by following your Astrodiet. Your ability to cut your losses, rebuild and start again, even when it pains you to do so, is the perfect qualification to become a successful slimmer.

It is understandable that you wish to lose weight and look your best because Scorpio is considered to be the sexiest sign of the zodiac. And if you're a typical Scorpio, you have a natural charisma and magnetic quality which makes others aware of your presence. You also possess the potent power to attract and hold others under your spell because they are intrigued and fascinated by you — all the more reason to refuse to allow your waistline to get out of control. Fortunately, your strong, resilient personality gives you the power to free yourself from those unwanted layers of surplus fat, so that the slim, vibrant, healthy you has the opportunity to emerge.

YOUR SLIMMING WEAKNESSES

One slimming obstacle which has probably caused you to pile on the pounds, is that your eating habits usually revolve around the most recent lifestyle you've adopted — according to what you are trying to prove at any particular time and what is going on in your life. Over the years you may have switched courses more than once where food's concerned. Whether your current diet consists mainly of convenience foods from the supermarket or a health shop special made up of a mixture of organically grown produce, ginseng and honey — it's obviously not keeping you slim, so it's time to change again. And this is one new beginning you'll be glad that you made, because any sexy Scorpio always likes to know that he or she is in peak condition.

MOOD MONITOR
Keep a record of your moods and the way you are feeling the next time you're tempted to raid the fridge. Whether it's boredom or depression that's eating at you, write it down and review your written analysis every week. The type of situation which threatens your peace of mind and therefore your figure, will soon become clear to you.

You can range from one extreme to another, from impressing others with your strong will, to depressing yourself with a sudden attack of self-indulgence. Life is rarely plain sailing for you, but many of the storms that can throw you off course are emotional in nature, because your feelings run especially deep. It is your extreme sensitivity to hurt and injustice that poses your greatest slimming obstacle as you never forget a grievance. And like the scorpion, with a barb in its tail which has the power to sting, you seek your revenge if someone treats you badly. Unfortunately, if you are denied the opportunity of dealing fairly and squarely with the person who has offended you, you are likely to give vent to your rage in another way — a way that is self-destructive — because you turn your body into your enemy by eating from anger rather than hunger.

Lack of challenge or of a worthwhile motivation represents

another potential threat to your figure. The feeling that your work, or your marriage or relationship, has no real direction or purpose can also cause you to attack food with a vengeance. Guard against allowing your life to become too boring or unrewarding even if this means creating incentives for yourself at those times when little is happening.

Another of your slimming weaknesses is your readiness to drive yourself on relentlessly, which can cause you to take drastic measures if you suddenly decide that you want to lose half a stone rapidly. It's possible you've tried to shed surplus pounds in the past by trying "crash" or extreme diet methods — you may have even fasted. As you discovered, these tactics always fail in the end.

Nothing is half-hearted with you, which makes it difficult for you to be moderate in your behaviour patterns. Your independent nature inclines you to be unwilling to confide all of your thoughts. This means that you often struggle alone with problems unnecessarily, when help and advice is available. It is not your way to give anything or anyone, including yourself, a second chance and at times, you can be altogether too inflexible. There is a stubborn, "fixed" side to your character which resists change. Be aware that this Scorpio personality trait could rob you of the success that is within your grasp, if you are forced to stray from your diet plan for any reason. As you know, you are not a person who is easily impressed or influenced, which in some ways is commendable. But be careful that you are not denying yourself the chance of profiting from other people's knowledge and experience.

DANGER GAMES

Don't neglect food awareness in your leisure moments, because you can easily become so absorbed in winning that hand of whist or Trivial Pursuit that it's not until after you've collected the kitty that you realise to your horror you've polished off a whole packet of cheese biscuits without noticing.

The specialist information already amassed in your Astrodiet and Astrocharts make it possible for you to diet safely and comfortably, knowing that you will ultimately measure up to your ideal size. The decision to "Slim by the Stars" is one that you'll never regret.

YOUR SLIMMING STRENGTHS

Mars and Pluto, the two powerful planets which rule your sign, are both associated with will-power and control. There's a part of you which has to win at all costs. Although at times this may not be to your advantage, it is a distinct point in your favour so far as slimming is concerned. Nothing is likely to stand in your way once you have set your sights on a new body-shape. You aim to be the boss, and usually are, so you're likely to resent food becoming more important to you than it should. Your healthy desire to rule your body with your mind, rather than allowing your stomach to be in charge, should be viewed as a valuable aid to dieting. It is only by controlling the amounts and the type of food that you eat, that you will be able to maintain your target weight once you have achieved it.

LOVE TO MAKE YOU FAT
Beware when the chance arises to linger over an intimate candle-lit dinner for two, as given the right company and the right atmosphere, the food tastes far better and the wine tastes far sweeter. And before you know it you could unwittingly eat enough for both of you, as your bathroom scales will tell you in no uncertain terms the next day.

You are tough, determined and resolute, so if you get your teeth into something, you rarely let go. When you start your slimming plan you fully expect to see it through to its completion, because you are one of those people who is unwilling to begin any project unless you seriously intend to stay with it — all the way. If by any chance you run into problems or your plans collapse, you have what it takes to pick up the pieces and start again, and you possess the courage, the tenacity and the strength of character to do so.

You will also appreciate the financial benefits that come from buying smaller quantities of food, as you are good with your cash and know how to obtain value for money by checking comparative prices and organising discounts. There's little that escapes your eagle eye and you scrutinise every detail of whatever's presented to you, working out all the implications and the possible rewards before proceeding. This means that you usually know exactly what you're letting yourself in for when you try something new — and are also able to identify the particular circumstances which have led you to becoming overweight.

You always feel more dynamic and ready to take on a new challenge if Mars is in your sign, or is in a position that favours Scorpio. These are the times to begin your diet, or restart it as necessary. Your "danger days" are when Mars is adversely placed in the heavens for Scorpio — days when you must pay extra attention to how you intend to keep yourself occupied. Also stay away from those people who make you upset or could cause you to eat or drink more than you should. The movements of Mars have been especially taken into account in the calculation of your Astrocharts.

YOU AND YOUR BODY

The reproductive organs and the pelvis are the parts of the body ruled by Scorpio. That is why your sign is linked with regeneration, sex and also the birth and death of the species.

Your ability to regenerate your own body stands you in good stead if ever your health is under par. You manage to draw on supplies of inner strength which help you fight off many of the everyday ailments that less resilient signs succumb to. Being a sensible weight for your size and knowing your appearance

> **BEGIN WITH A BLITZ**
> *Channel the all-or-nothing energy that marks out the Scorpio by dealing with any chaos in your surroundings. Take your mind off hunger pangs on a Danger day by having an all-out tidying blitz on wardrobes and cupboards*

isn't letting you down is especially important for you, because your body, health and eating patterns are always strongly influenced by your moods and the state of your mind.

Your forceful energy needs to be channelled correctly for you to stay on top form, as you can suffer from extremes of weight if you are not motivated to stay with your diet. That is why it pays you to include regular energetic physical exercise in your daily programme. Those Scorpios who are sports orientated will gravitate towards competitive games, as the chance to win while you're letting off steam suits your determined personality. You may also be champion at one or more of the martial arts, such as judo or karate. However if you are one of those Scorpios who loathes sport, you'll be happy to know that digging the garden, a lively spate of housework, or polishing the car, will serve equally well to tone you up and keep you in shape, by burning up some of your excess calories and energy. Remember there's no need to punish your body in your fight against your flab: walking briskly or swimming are also excellent alternative forms of exercise.

Touch and body contact mean a lot to you as a sensual Scorpio, so you'll especially benefit from a soothing massage whenever you're feeling tense or need to unwind. An ideal massage for you is the type used in aromatherapy, where essential oils are matched to your particular personality type. If your budget doesn't run to a professional treatment don't despair. You can do yourself a lot of good by smoothing on a body-balm, all over, to relax your muscles gently after a hot shower or bath. Treating your skin to loving care, from day one of your diet, will help avoid stretch marks appearing as your store cupboard of fatty flesh gradually disappears.

SCORPIO SPECIAL
In your heart, you'd like to keep your diet a secret. So it's as well that your Water sign diet asks you to give just one week over to serious slimming — and allows for packed lunches. On some days after that, you can eat normally, but not 'over the top'. No-one need know your plan until the pounds have slipped away and your new measurements bring admiration. The dramatic ending that Scorpios adore!

As Scorpio is a Water sign, you should regard water as the liquid that nature intends you to drink. Not only does it add to that full-up feeling, it is non-fattening, inexpensive and cleanses and purifies your system. Why not pour out a glass of the fizzy mineral sort for yourself and sip it before and in-between your meals?

YOU AND YOUR EMOTIONS

Although Scorpio is a sign associated with sex, many Scorpios stay unmarried. The fear of making a mistake and being hurt can be even stronger than the passions that burn up inside you. If only your fat cells would burn up in the same way! You seek written guarantees in love as you need to know that your chosen one will have eyes only for you and be faithful to you forever. And if they're not, you're sure to find out. You possess an uncanny knack of being able to detect the truth — as others learn to their cost if they've tried to cover up their actions with lies or excuses. You even manage to ferret out things you're not supposed to know. And just to be totally infuriating, you somehow manage to keep your own secrets carefully hidden.

You have a powerful capacity to love and protect those you care about. You are passionate, loyal and a person of commitment. You need to feel very close to your partner in a relationship. Ideally they must be ready to take you seriously — your ambitions, your talents, your priorities — and most importantly, your principles. Apart from all this they must be as self-motivated as you are and very gutsy, because if there's one thing you can't abide, it's someone whom you consider to be a weak, spineless character. Even with this quite short shopping list, you can begin to understand why some of your fellow Scorpios stay single, often travelling a lonely road in life, not realising that they have passed by more than one potentially suitable partner in their endless search for perfection. Whether or not you are happily matched, be aware that demanding too much from another human being and refusing to accept their failings can only result in disenchantment, which can be one of the root causes of overweight problems for you.

Once you've accepted the initial differences between you and the Fire sign people (their lack of subtlety when they want something, and their different emotional needs), you'll discover that there are many similarities. Both of you are fairly dynamic and ambitious and also self-motivated. The spirit of adventure that burns within all Fire people is attractive to you as well as their ability to see the bright side of life. One of the things that they like about you is that you're a challenge. It can take them forever to figure you out — if they ever do. A Fire partner or friend makes an ideal slimming companion for you because their eagerness to see results, which will keep them dieting on come what may, is the encouragement you need to prove that you're a winner too.

A relationship with someone born under one of the three Earth signs, Taurus, Virgo or Capricorn, could satisfy many of your needs, because like you, they are security conscious and work to a plan of campaign. However, Earth people regard food as one of the prime sources of security, so tend to offer edible gifts for anniversaries and as tokens of their appreciation. Even so, they respond positively to logic and commonsense, so your Earth companions will be supportive to your slimming efforts if you point out the numerous benefits you and they, if applicable, can gain from losing weight.

There is a natural flow between you and other Water people, Scorpios like yourself or Cancer or Pisces. They will calm you down when you're het up, comfort you in times of trouble and help you relax. You always feel comfortable and at ease in the presence of a Water friend or spouse, because you are both very sensitive and intuitive. This means that you stand a good chance of enjoying wedded bliss together, and you both seek permanency in a relationship. Your mutual empathy can also be of great value in a joint slimming effort, as you will sense when each other is in the mood to nibble — and also know the precise preventative measures to take for the circumstances, besides what to say to boost each other's morale, if the bathroom scales have registered disappointment.

The Air people — Gemini, Libra and Aquarius — go about dealing with life's problems in a entirely different way to you. They are thinkers, who analyse and question everything, including their own emotions. They are firm believers in mind over matter — brain cells over fat cells — and are often at odds with themselves as their passions and feelings tend to be suppressed or regarded as irrational. This will reinforce your own desire to take control of your weight. Together, you make an unlikely couple, but it can work out if you find a common cause and allow each other to have a certain amount of independence. Even so, you would have to curb your Scorpionic possessiveness as all Air people need the right to flit away occasionally, without being asked too many questions.

YOUR CREATIVE ENERGIES

Scorpios are known for their nose for a mystery and ability to investigate and find what is hidden. This gift may draw you to hobbies which involve research or detective work. Collecting antiques and archeology are classic Scorpio type interests. You also adore a competition or a puzzle. Most Scorpios play cards, chess, dominos or other socially orientated games.

Discovery holidays were made for you because they provide the means to roll a challenge and an adventure into one glorious experience. Wherever you go, you need to explore and satisfy yourself that you have seen all there is to see and also spotted what less observant signs have overlooked.

Similar to those born under the other Water signs, you love music in all its forms and are also drawn to the arts and literature. You expect to spend a lot of your leisure time on your own, but it is actually good for you to choose a few spare-time activities that you can share with others. Not only are you a good listener, but you can also make a valuable contribution to any debate. Your social style leans towards intimate get-togethers, especially twosomes or rendezvous with a few tried and tested friends. While you will attend or give a large party if there's a good reason to do so, you are happiest in the cosy companionship of a small group. When it's your turn to entertain others, you do so, like so much of your life, with careful thought and planning. This means you can follow your diet allowances without any real problems. It is when the boot's on the other foot and someone's is taking you out, that you must be on your guard.

DON'T HIDE SEXINESS
When it comes to fashion, your sign and style is associated with all that is downright sexy. Don't let surplus pounds allow you to hide inside drab, muted tones or dowdy styles. For now, use bright and attention-getting accessories. And while you slim away the inches, plan how you'll buy an outfit to knock 'em cold when you reach your target weight.

You can be a dedicated do-it-yourselfer, ready to tackle anything, from hanging wallpaper to laying a parquet floor. You prefer to have a purpose and a goal in sight when you allocate your time and energy to a spare-time activity. You soon get stuck in to your latest enthusiasm, once you're sure what's required — a fact which will help you make a positive start to your diet and exercise regime. You put your heart and soul into any project you undertake, so need to find gratifying outlets for your creative energies.

Renovation is your forte, whether that's a modest touch of 'make-do-and-mend' or something more ambitious, such as rebuilding an engine or restoring a priceless work of art. As you are rarely daunted, you often take pleasure in tackling projects that others consider impossible. This means that no matter how much weight you have to shift, you'll do it. You are capable and resourceful and thoroughly enjoy pitting your wits against a problem. Never forget that Scorpio is associated with birth and death and one of the most powerful signs in the zodiac. The regenerative forces that flow through you will help you now to let old ways of life die and new ones begin — so that you can enjoy every day in the best of health, knowing you look as good as you feel.

SAGITTARIUS

November 22 — December 21

Sagittarius, which is the ninth sign of the zodiac, is symbolised by the mythological Centaur - half man and half beast, which represents the struggle between the base instincts of Man and the aspirations of the higher self. Jupiter, the ruler of Sagittarius, takes twelve years to complete its journey through the zodiac; many Sagittarians experience a pattern of important life changes every twelve years. Jupiter is associated with expansion and considered to bring good fortune, giving those born under this Fire sign a strong belief in their own good luck and regular opportunities to make their dreams come true.

YOUR SLIMMING CHARACTER

As a Sagittarian, you make a very good dieting subject because your eternal optimism makes you believe in your own success. Your expansive attitudes extend to all areas of your life, which you intend to live to the full. This will encourage you to set your sights high in slimming. However it is only too easy for those ruled by the planet of growth, Jupiter, to do so literally and spread out — overloading their bodies with extra weight as the years roll on. The movement of Jupiter has been taken into account in your Astrochart as both your weight and your spirits tend to rise when this friendly planet is in a part of the heavens where it influences Sagittarians.

You firmly believe in tomorrow but must guard against under-valuing what is readily available or what is happening in the present. As a perpetual schemer and planner, one who is ready to make changes and take chances, you will have to accept that retaining a weight loss is only possible by eating wisely on a daily basis. You, in particular, must make healthy eating the rule rather than the exception.

YOUR SLIMMING WEAKNESSES

Many Sagittarians are impulsive eaters and there's no doubt that you like the spice of life. In your book this includes exotic dishes as well as those tempting sticky cream cakes, nuts and savoury snacks which are piled high with calories. Your main slimming weakness is that moderation doesn't often enter your thoughts — you tend to do everything in a big way.

Your gregarious nature and generosity says "stop and have another helping" or "have another drink" to your guests. All too often you consume glasses of wine, beer or refreshing bottles of fizz which contain large quantities of sugar, which, in turn, converts to unwanted fat. It's imperative to differentiate between need and desire and take a firm line with yourself if you realise that the latter is your true motivation for helping yourself to drinks and nibbles in between meals.

Another of your slimming obstacles is that inner restlessness which can cause you to abandon a scheme before you have really given it a fair trial. In fact you can roar ahead too quickly for your own good. Although you usually know when the right time has come to act, you sometimes allow success to slip through your fingers by failing to follow through or to wait for results. It's essential to be one hundred per cent behind your diet plan to become slim and stay that way. If you are single-minded about achieving your required weight loss, you will soon be wearing the size of clothes you know you should be wearing: and you'll be thankful you made the effort.

ABROAD VIEW

In many lands, you only have to look around and study the shape of the native population to establish that their traditional fare, as tempting as it is, is very fattening. Satisfy your taste for the unusual by rationing your experimental eating to those delicious foreign fruits and crunchy local salads — without too much oil.

Your innermost yearning is to travel — to pack a suitcase at a moment's notice and go off, even if it's just for a weekend away with friends. You have a yearning to explore the world, new places, new faces and also new foods. Unfortunately, this doesn't always go hand in hand with watching your weight. When you are away from your home, make up your mind to be doubly diet-conscious. Curb your weakness for interesting looking sauces —

which add inches as well as flavour — and opt for grilled fish and meat.

Holidays are very important to you, so you shouldn't deny yourself the chance to pack a suitcase and take off when the opportunity arises, as it's good for you to have different surroundings from time to time, even if just for the occasional weekend. But be aware that exotic flavours and sauces are always suspect. The average shape of the local population should provide you with an insight into the fattening potential of the traditional fare.

YOUR SLIMMING STRENGTHS

In many ways you are a born gambler because you are naturally adventurous and ready to try anything once. You will be happy to be the first in your circle to try this new way of slimming. You usually throw yourself into a new project with a speed and a confidence that leaves others standing. This self-assurance and eagerness to see results is one of your greatest slimming strengths and will soon help you realise the dreams you hold of achieving your perfect weight.

Like the other two Fire signs, Aries and Leo, you possess a certain quality of energy and enthusiasm which is directed in whatever you do. The shopping, the cooking, the measuring out — you'll take all of these in your stride with such vigour that you'll be hard pushed to find time to sit down and enjoy your daily allowance of food and drink. The supermarket will become a whole new world to you.

You also love to learn and love to share what you have learned with others. This has earned you the well-deserved reputation of

TROLLEY BUST
Instead of racing around with a trolley scooping up panic buys of convenience food (due to that impulsive invitation you gave to a few friends or neighbours "to come around to my place for a bite to eat?") Work from a shopping list and study comparative food values. Just think of the benefits to your cash-flow: as you lose pounds of weight, you'll save pounds in money.

being the teacher of the zodiac. And as soon as you realise that your diet really works, you will be anxious to share the secret of your success and diet plan with your overweight friends or family. You're unlikely to be considered a diet bore because your sense of humour and amusing way of telling a tale will make others eager to listen to your slimming saga — they'll anxiously wait for the next instalment. Your bubbly enthusiasm will encourage them to follow your shining, and slimming, example. Another advantage of talking about your weight-reducing plan is that it will strengthen your own conviction that it's the only sensible way of life for you to lead.

If you are a typical Sagittarian, you are at your happiest when you are busily planning for the future and you possess a breadth of vision which allows you clearly to identify your main objective and "go for it". This ability to visualise and believe in tomorrow is another valuable slimming strength — one that will assist your battle with overweight. Imagine yourself the shape and the size that you would like to be as this is an important step towards making your wishes come true.

FIT FOR ANYTHING

Try to exercise every day, if necessary snatching a few minutes here and a few minutes there. The motto for you is NEVER put off until tomorrow the press-ups or brisk walk that matters today. An exercise bike or a rowing machine will help you to fight the flab and also keep your circulation toned up.

Once you have risen to a challenge, you are not easily discouraged. It's probably true to say that you need a challenge to bring out the best in you as you love to prove you can win. Few put in as much effort as you do once you've set an ambition. Make your next ambition one that will benefit your health as well as your morale: the ambition to be a smaller size, the one that you would most prefer to buy clothes for.

You are naturally competitive, so can cope with the challenge of changing your eating patterns. In this campaign you have the ideal prize waiting to be collected, a prize you can keep with you for the rest of your life — the secret of looking good and feeling fantastic. There is an honesty and a frankness about your personality that both pleases and offends others. You won't bat an eyelid about telling your host or hostess that their chocolate gateau is "for fatties only"; fortunately you usually manage to make people laugh when you are outspoken, so are easily forgiven. This forthrightness is an asset in your fight against flab because you will not feel intimidated into saying "Yes" to a helping of fat-making dessert, when it's the last thing you need.

YOU AND YOUR BODY

The hips, bottom and thighs are the parts of the body particularly associated with Sagittarius. Pay attention to yours because they usually supply you with a clear indication when it's time to go on a diet. Suddenly it becomes obvious that you've collected wobbly fat and unwanted inches on your bottom and the tops of your legs — more than on any other parts of your body — while your waistline appears to be expanding by the minute.

Your remarkable capacity to enjoy life means that you tend to be a fairly healthy sign. Your weight problems, as well as general ailments, are often linked with the lack of a worthwhile challenge, so you should take steps to ensure that your existence never becomes too humdrum or uneventful.

The great outdoors represents the perfect exercise ground for you, whether you're sporting a bat and ball or jogging round the park. The community sports centre is also ideal Sagittarian territory, but it has to be your decision to enrol because you are not easily led. As it's a top priority on your list to be mobile — by land, sea or air — owning a car is usually an essential part of the Sagittarian budget.

As the adventurers of the zodiac, you need excitement and should be out and about exploring and broadening your horizons. Sitting moping in front of the television for long periods is definitely bad news for you. Favour healthy, out of doors activities, such as camping, walking, ball games or boating, which will keep the roses in your cheeks and act like a tonic for your health. Also explore the keep fit activities that are available close to home, such as your local sports or health centre. Welcome any chance to immerse yourself in a new interest.

The busy pace of your life can sometimes, however, place a tremendous strain on you and it may not be until you feel totally

FUEL FOR THOUGHT

Put as much careful thought into the choice of fuel for your body as you normally put to the fuel you buy for your car, even if it means that you must change the habits of a lifetime and throw your store of chocolate bars and savoury nibbles out of the window. It's pointless knowing that you're really a lively, sleek, racing model if other people look at you and think that you're built like a tank!

exhausted, that you sit back and realise that your body is looking neglected and the worse for wear. It's then that your brutal honesty with yourself pays dividends, as you stand in front of a full length mirror and shock horror sets in.

Although you're usually an active person and may even be athletic, you need to relax whenever possible and ease out of the fast lane. Stress can set in and store up in your back and shoulders. Frustration and anxiety can also cause you to feel stressed, particularly if your talents are not being stretched to the full. The key to your healthy living and success as a slimmer is to find an interesting channel for your energies and keep a check on how your body is standing up to the hammering you often give it. Once you are physically back on form and in shape, don't allow yourself to slip back into bad habits. Eat to stay slim and make it a long-term commitment.

YOU AND YOUR EMOTIONS

Companionship is an essential part of love to you, so your partner must also be your very best friend. Warm, affectionate and energetic, you need someone who is as adventurous and independent as you. They must also accept your restless nature and the prime urge you have to be your own person and follow your own star. Most importantly, they must know how to let their hair down and have fun, as the ability to laugh and enjoy life together, and even slim together, is the formula for a successful relationship for you.

Your sunny, outgoing disposition attracts others instantly. It doesn't take long for your amiable approach and sense of humour to break down the barriers of others, even those who are stuffy or reserved. Other people fascinate you, so you will go out of your way to meet someone who sounds interesting. You love to cheer

SNAP HAPPY

Take a photograph of yourself now, bulges and all, and then another each week, to supply pictorial evidence of how you're doing. Your photos will make it clear to you when you've achieved your ideal weight. With the help of your Astrodiets and charts you can stay that way.

other people up and give them encouragement when they're depressed, so one of the fringe benefits of slimming, so far as you're concerned, will be the positive effect on the friends you have who are unhappily overweight.

Many look at you and assume that you haven't a care in the world because you rarely confide your deepest feelings to anyone, not even the one who knows you the best. Nevertheless, there's a very sensitive, romantic person hiding behind that breezy exterior. If you're true to your sign you are something of a dreamer, an incurable idealist, and a total softy at heart. You'll be the first to crack a joke about your diet intentions but deep down, you're well aware of the serious reasons behind your need to get to grips with your surplus weight .You know, instinctively, that fat slows you down, looks unsightly and that it can also put a strain on your heart.

As you are a person who thrives on change, it is easy for you to become dissatisfied once you take love for granted. Your endless search for excitement can often be the root cause of domestic squabbles and emotional upsets. Recognise the need you have for constant action; without it you become restless, bored and tend to eat. Your diet plan is designed with your active type of personality in mind.

A relationship with another Fire sign person, a Sagittarian like yourself, a Leo or an Aries, should provide you with the stimulus you demand, as they share your hankering to be at the hub of the activity. Although you can both be extravagant and are likely to challenge each other, another Fire person can handle your directness and occasional lack of subtlety and may even appreciate the fact that they know where they stand. You look at life in the same way as they do, with the belief that everything you want will be yours eventually. As a slimming companion, you couldn't do better, because both of you are set on winning and this double helping of determination is enough to ensure that together you'll achieve your targets without compromising on a single pound.

It's a completely different story when it comes to you and a Water person, someone born under the signs of Cancer, Scorpio or Pisces. These people are highly sensitive and emotional, with a tendency to take things personally. Even a light-hearted comment, such as "Are you eating for two?" when you see your Water colleague or spouse diving into a bag of sweets or a bag of crisps, is enough to provoke an angry response or even worse, a hurt silence. In a marriage partnership, you may find it hard to cope with a Water sign's constant need for reassurance of your undying love and affection, while they can feel threatened by your impulsiveness and quick temper. Even so, they will be ready to calm you down when you're het up and to listen to your problems, offering support and back-up — even if means putting themselves out. In return, you are the perfect pal for an overweight Water-baby because your ability to tell others what's good for them will soon have them sold on the idea that an astrologically based slimming plan makes sense.

You should relate especially well to anyone born under an Air sign, a Gemini, Libra or Aquarius. Although Air people possess a certain coolness and detachment about them and you, as a Fire person, are warm, ardent and above all, enthusiastic, together you make a good combination. They will appreciate your fiery strengths and not be unduly bothered about your weaknesses, while you will adore free thinking and often witty conversation. For this reason you benefit from dieting with an Air person who will soon have you looking forward to the times you eat or exercise together.

Joining forces with an Earth person, a Taurus, Virgo or Capricorn, could bring security into your life. The very nature of Earth people is to seek lasting qualities, to stabilise and put down roots. Your bold approach to life and willingness to take a risk, if the occasion demands it, will help an Earth partner to make the most of their own opportunities. At the same time, your drive and positive manner will provide the necessary boost for them to slim. They will find it hard to comprehend your desire to wander and experiment, but they are realistic enough to accept that that's the way you are. You can learn from their structured way of dealing with problems and see where you should slow down. An Earth partner will encourage you to stick to your diet plan and also to eat your slimming meals in the correct order and one day at a time!

YOUR CREATIVE ENERGIES

You love speed. Do you remember as a child wanting to shoot ahead on your bicycle or skate board and be faster than everyone else? As an adult you may still hanker after a fast car so you can zoom off into the sunset whenever the mood grabs you. This risk-taking element within you, the part of you that quite enjoys dancing with danger, is your creative force, surging up within you, searching for an outlet. Unfortunately, a weight reducing plan is one thing that shouldn't be hurried, so you now need patience and perseverance, two qualities that rarely come easily to those born under your sign

You are an entertaining story-teller and make an excellent show-biz personality and a scintillating sales-person as you excel in front of an audience. Your personality thrives on any kind of group activity — this can assist you now, especially if it's up to you to encourage others to stay with their dieting plans. Enthusing your friends serves to reinforce your own intentions.

You pour a lot of your creative energy into your social life and can always come up with a novel idea on where to go for an outing. You understand the true party spirit and want others to enjoy themselves as much as you do. If at all possible, you should join up with friends and swap humorous dieting experiences and one-upmanship progress reports.

Although you may enjoy redesigning the kitchen or hanging pictures down the full stretch of the wall, a quiet stay at home would

WATCH OUT!
Be aware of what you're drinking when you dine out or socialise. In one fell swoop, alcohol adds calories without nutrients, stimulates your appetite and manages to dull your senses, so that your resolve weakens. Limit your drinks and you'll keep a clear head — the morning after as well — plus the satisfaction that you've completed another day of your Astrodiet plan successfully.

soon make you feel caged in and stifled. You need to be able to get up and take off on impulse, so you rarely visit the same holiday location twice. Your suitcase is probably well used and though you may forget to pack sensible walking shoes or an umbrella, you rarely forget your camera as you derive additional pleasure from showing your photographs of those action-packed and memorable moments you've had.

Whether you are young or old you possess a great zest for life and seldom hesitate to involve yourself in new activities. You are versatile and ready to have a go at anything, which is why you can be multi-talented. The shadow side of this image is seen in the Sagittarians who are over-optimistic about their ability to deliver and disperse their energies in many different directions, thereby failing to become proficient at anything. Learning to invest your time carefully is the most certain way for you to find success, so don't stray from your diet plan, as this is one time when you should make up your mind to stay totally single minded.

Your optimism and desire to see resultys will stand you in good stead to achieve your desired weight reduction — knowing that you have also established the healthy eating patterns that can provide you with the necessary energy to live life to the full in true Sagittarian style.

CAPRICORN

December 22 — January 19

Although the constellation of Capricorn, the tenth sign of the zodiac, is not especially easy to locate in the heavens, it was regarded by the ancient astrologers as a very sacred sign, because it governs the period, in the Northern hemisphere, when the nights begin to shorten. Ruled by Saturn, a planet related to structure, Capricorns possess a strong urge to instil order into their surroundings. The sure-footed Goat which is able to climb to the top of the highest mountain is the symbol of Capricorn and those born under this sign are considered to be careful and ambitious.

YOUR SLIMMING CHARACTER

Capricorn is traditionally the sign of the establishment and associated with government, law and order, so it is natural for you to seek a set of rules for your life. In fact, when you were a child, you may have been especially conscientious. When you think back, do you remember being put in charge of your brothers or sisters to keep an eye on what they were up to? The answer's almost certainly "yes", because even little Capricorns have an air of authority and know how to take control. Even as an adult, you are usually happiest when you have recognisable guide-lines to follow, which makes you a superb candidate for an organised slimming programme. The written instructions, the carefully calculated Astrocharts, the planned diets and the do's and the don'ts, are exactly the style of language that any law-abiding Capricorn appreciates.

It is a mistake for others to assume you are unadventurous or afraid of change, because this is not at all the case. But you do prefer to think things through thoroughly, rather than acting on impulse. Although you look to the future, you also value tradition and the past. Once you have done your homework and made a decision, you can leave others standing because like the Goat (usually a nifty mover) which symbolises your sign, you have what it takes to travel fast and arrive safely. You now have the chance to be nimble and agile — all the more reason to stick to your diet, especially as it's unacceptable to your image to climb a flight of stairs panting for breath. Many of your fellow Capricorns go right to the top of their chosen occupations, because yours is the sign of the planner and the builder.

YOUR SLIMMING WEAKNESSES

Conservation is a key factor in your life because Capricorns are the protectors and preservers of inherited resources and traditions. You may be acutely interested in restoring old buildings, or a leading light in the ecology movement, but even if you're not, it's likely that you place great store in the customs you've grown up with, and refuse to make change purely for the sake of it. This represents your greatest slimming obstacle, because it is your old way of eating that has padded you out.

ALERT TO DANGER
Learn awareness eating, which means never nibbling as a side-line when you're doing something else. In the past the pounds could have crept on without you noticing while you were quietly reading or watching television, so always set a table or tray and sit down to concentrate on your food, so your brain registers that you've had a proper meal.

The fact that you are now unhappy with the way you look, makes it obvious that the time has come to adopt a brand new lifestyle — one that is based not on old fashioned ideas, but on current knowledge about the body and the way it stores fat. No longer can you afford to base your eating patterns on what your stomach has learned to expect. It is by acquiring a new set of eating habits which allow you to balance your calorie intake with your energy output that you will be able to lose weight and know that you can stay slim.

You possess an excellent sense of timing, but this can be a two-edged sword when it comes to slimming, especially if you are in the habit of taking frequent breaks for refreshments. Your body-clock will continue to ring its alarm bells, to tell you it's time for your tea and toast, or coffee and cakes, until you have reset it to your new timetable, the one that fits in with your slim style of eating. Munch on a stick of celery or a small apple to appease any unsatisfied feeling you have in the early days of dieting and it will not be long before you will be able to do without eating in-between meals.

Yet another potential slimming problem for your sign is the Saturnine or "heavy", serious side to the Capricorn personality. This can sometimes make you look on the gloomy side of life and impose unnecessary limitations on yourself. A deep-rooted Capricorn idea that needs examining is your own conviction that you were fated to carry a heavy load in life. (Although this is exactly what you're now doing, literally, in the form of the fat distributed in generous layers around your midriff, hips and thighs).

Feeling low or dispirited acts like a brake on your dieting, especially if your will-power starts to show the slightest signs of weakening. Guard against trying to compensate for an aching heart, a disappointment or simply a feeling of being "down", with a pick-me-up in the shape of a box of chocolates or a packet of savouries. Your Astrochart will warn you well in advance when an attack of the proverbial blues could strike, giving you the chance to immerse yourself in those interests which cheer you up and give you fat-free pleasure.

Many Capricorns lack confidence in their earlier years and wait until the second part of their lives to realise the dreams of their youth. Whatever your age, don't stand in your own path now, especially as it's highly probable that in the past, you have often encouraged others to succeed in projects related to self-improvement. Take your own sensible advice to resolve your overweight problem and make the very next date on your Astrochart the day to start your action.

TRICK AND TREAT
Here's another trick of the slimming trade that will give you a head start in the war against weight-gain. Fill your plate up with fewer calories, so that you feel you've eaten normal rations. A little food goes a long way if you use modern kitchen aids. Set your slicing machine on THIN for cucumber, onions or potatoes and use a fine grater for cheese or carrot. If you follow this method, two ounces will turn into a really satisfing-looking mound of appetising nosh

YOUR SLIMMING STRENGTHS

Whether you are male or female, your ideal image as a Capricorn is elegant and sophisticated. Your natural awareness of how you look is a definite plus factor for your slimming ambitions. The awful thought that you could be described as a "corpulent Capricorn" will motivate you to set your sights high and persevere with your dieting — right until the day that your tape measure smiles its approval.

It's that ambitious streak within you which drives you on until you achieve exactly what you set out to do. You are willing to accept responsibility and will even practice self-denial in the pursuit of your objectives. In fact, you have the ideal weapons to assure victory in your fight against flab.

Your grit and determination are two of your most positive slimming strengths. In common with the other two Earth signs, Taurus and Virgo, you also possess a typically "down to earth" quality, which helps you to keep your feet on the ground and stand strong if ever the going starts to get tough. This means you will be able to achieve the weight and size that is right for you. You are not concerned with scoring points over other slimmers and are not arrogant, so are willing to learn from other people's experiences and stand to profit from the professional advice offered in your Astrodiet — created with you in mind.

> **TO GRIPS WITH GREENS**
> *In the Earth sign diet, salads and green vegetables are yours in unlimited quantities. But it's up to you to make them interesting - that's where your Capricorn mix of organisation and imagination comes in. Buy small, frequent quantities of the new greens increasingly available in the shops — Chinese leaves? Snow or snap peas? Bean sprouts? Radicchio lettuce? —and enjoy the experimenting.*

You are not one of life's gamblers and are not one to be over-impressed with promises of quick and spectacular weight losses. It has taken you a long time, possibly years, to become overweight, so if you try to slim too quickly you can expect your body to put up strong resistance. Losing weight gradually ensures that the pounds lost aren't regained the moment you ease up a little. Fortunately, it was probably a Capricorn who first said that "if it's worth having, it's worth waiting for" because you are very realistic and extremely patient. This patience is a wonderful Capricorn slimming strength, which will allow you to reduce in size at a steady and sensible speed. You prefer to see constant progress on a diet which doesn't deplete your energies, upset your routine or make you feel hungry all the time.

You'll be pleased to know that your Astrodiet will gently and persistently remove that stubborn fatty tissue which looks so unsightly. Did you know that it is important to keep your survival mechanism under control to slim successfully? The way to do this is to eat slightly less than your daily calorific requirements, without cutting back on the essential vitamins, mineral salts and other nutrients that your body needs to be efficient. Crash diets never work because they cause ravenous hunger and slow down your body's functions.

The sheer economic sense of buying smaller quantities of food, food which is high in nourishment, will appeal to you as most Capricorns have a shrewd head for business, often acting as the financial counsellor to others. Do you find that you instinctively save for that proverbial "rainy day" even when money is short? Your thriftiness and sensible attitudes towards spending will help you resist buying impulse foods which are surplus to your requirements.

Your gift for quiet concentration and your readiness to do the groundwork before you make your moves, makes you a winner in the slimming stakes. You tend to

AFTER YOU'VE SINNED

Capricorns can be unrelenting taskmasters, making life hard for themselves as much as for others. When your diet has slipped - as it may, on a Danger Day - you must learn to forgive yourself. Just cut down a little on the following day. Simply cut out the 'treat' that you are allowed. But resist strongly the urge to punish yourself by embarking on a total fast.

be particularly single-minded when Saturn, your planetary ruler, is in a complementary position in the heavens to your own sign. As you will find it easier to achieve your desired weight loss if you start off at the most favourable time, the daily aspects of Saturn have been taken into account in the calculation of your Astrocharts.

YOU AND YOUR BODY

If you're a typical Capricorn, you are keenly interested in the workings of your body, so are ready to take positive action to put matters right if ever you become aware, or even faintly suspicious, that all is not well. The second part of a Capricorn's life is usually when the snuffles, coughs and chills of their childhood, teens and twenties are firmly behind them. Whether you are enjoying the first flush of youth or looking forward to retirement, you will appreciate the need to stay healthy and in good shape to enjoy the full benefits that you, as a Capricorn, can derive from maturity.

Your bones, especially your knees, are the parts of your anatomy that are associated with Capricorn, so make a point of doing those kind of exercises which keep you supple as part of a daily limbering-up routine. Yours is a fairly physical sign, so make regular keep fit sessions as much of a habit as brushing your teeth — but gently does it — stay within your capability and avoid feeling worn out.

Your body will also benefit from another healthy habit, one that is low in cost and especially relevant if you're a "night owl". You should firmly resist eating your main meal late at night because it takes longer to burn calories up once you've "switched off" and gone to sleep. Food eaten immediately prior to bed-time stands far more chance of being filed away as fat. (It may interest you to know that you use only about 30 calories an hour once you are asleep — the amount supplied by a very small apple.)

Laughter is your greatest tonic and a powerful preventative medicine against illness, as well as a boost for you as a would be slimmer. Being over-concerned with the worries of the world and other people's problems, as well as your own, can weigh you down and depress you, sometimes

LOGGING THE LOSSES

Capricorns have a strong sense of family history. So now's the chance to start a 'slimming journal' that might, one day, be an inspiration to your children. Note your weight, week by week. Especially note how it varies between the 'two weeks of strict dieting' and the 'four weeks of moderation' that add up to your Earth sign diet. Remember to add dates, notes about prices, events, even the weather — you are creating a piece of history driving you to find consolation of the edible kind — you may still be carrying the evidence of your last bout of worrying around your waistline.

In common with Taureans and Virgos, the other two Earth signs, you tend to follow habitual patterns of eating and drinking. This means that you may now have to rethink many of your long established ideas about food. Particularly if you are a member of an overweight family. Your excess pounds are more likely to be the effects of overloading your plate for years than due to glandular reasons. It's to your advantage to familiarise yourself with your correct diet plan well before your next family reunion.

YOU AND YOUR EMOTIONS

It is likely that there are certain similarities between your approach to love and your approach to slimming because you are deliberate and realistic about your emotional needs. Although hearts and flowers are not necessarily your style, you seek a deep and meaningful emotional relationship and regard marriage, or a long-term commitment, as a natural development. You rarely give your heart completely unless there's a contract for life offered in return. It doesn't take you long to make up your mind when you meet someone who is a potential partner, even if you choose to keep them guessing or at arm's length for a while. Having a clear structure or framework is as important to you in your love-life as in your diet and fitness plan, because you like to know all the rules, the chances of success and the possible future developments, in whatever you do.

Ideally your partner should share your long-term ambitions, your practical approach to life and be reliable, resourceful, but wildly exciting! He or she should also have the ability to bring out your delightful sense of humour which is sometimes lost on those who judge by first impressions. You can be wonderfully romantic, in fact more romantic than some would believe possible. Underneath that self-disciplined and sensible exterior, there's a passionate heart ticking away, but the defensive barrier you put up if you're uncertain of someone's intentions can make you appear cool, even icy and indifferent. Although you tend to be a very self-contained person, don't be too distant now, because you could miss out on the encouragement and support of your friends and family — who may even like to diet along with you.

You relate well to those born under the Water signs, Cancer, Scorpio and Pisces, because this is a non-competitive and mutually supportive combination, which will work well in both business and emotional relationships. Once a Water friend or relative decides to help you slim, they will do everything in their power to help you, even if that means eating stringently themselves, in order to stop you feeling that you're missing out. However, as caring and loving as your Water companions are, don't accept a Water person's hospitality unless they have been told you're on a diet because their basic urge is to feed and look after others.

The Fire sign people, Aries, Leos and Sagittarius, can add an element of excitement to your life but their liking for action and desire to proceed at a fast pace may sometimes prove rather taxing for your nerves and composure. The Fire personality is usually fairly assertive but doesn't always appreciate that what's right for them may not always necessarily be right for others. Having said that, a Fire partner makes a wonderful slimming ally because even if no word is spoken, they will make you feel incredibly guilty, just by the way that they look at you, whenever you reach for that biscuit tin or an extra helping of a particularly delicious dinner.

The Air people, Gemini, Libra and Aquarians, are always receptive to the winds of change, so if you hope to tempt an Air sign into joining you in slimming, sell them the thought that you are ready to give a new way of eating a try. A long-term partnership with an Air person requires effort and understanding on both parts because while you prefer to see one project through at a time, another bonus point for a potential slimmer, in the Air person's book it is quite O.K. to change direction at the drop of a hat — or to fly off at a tangent. As you can see, this could present its fair share of problems.

Life with another Earth sign, Taurus, Virgo or a fellow Capricorn, will be fairly predictable and very organised. You will find many things to agree about, so this relationship can work well — providing you are allowed to make your own decisions. Always bear in mind that as the cardinal Earth sign you are a leader, so are unlikely to find true fulfilment with anyone who holds you back or constantly questions your movements. Where slimming's concerned, this could be a successful combination. An Earth companion shares your methodical approach to a problem, so you will be able to back each other up with dozens of practical reasons for losing weight, if ever one of you is waivering.

YOUR CREATIVE ENERGIES

Many fine musicians, potters, sculptors, artists and architects are born under your sign because while many of the more flamboyant signs are spouting out their ideas with heated enthusiasm, you are quietly turning dreams into reality, words into books and blueprints into buildings.

You recognise that a work of art is usually nine tenths hard work and one tenth inspiration. Whatever you do, you apply yourself with tremendous determination. As you are also constructive and persevering, you often excel in more than one leisure activity. You dislike wasting time on being idle, so it is to be expected that you want to put your off-duty moments to good use. You will, therefore, also

SAFETY MEASURES
Your Danger days will be easier to survive if you cultivate the company of those who are either young in years or young at heart. Youthful people usually hold the key to the child within you — the child who eats only when it is hungry and who knows how to play. Gemini, Aries and Sagittarius will all help you to have a good laugh, relax a little and forget about food for a while.

regard time spent on body-care and exercise as worthwhile. Although you possess as many dreams as anyone else, you differentiate between fantasy and reality, so usually manage to develop your creative talents to the full.

It is certain that you will have taken the trouble to become something of an authority on any subject that holds your interest. This thoroughness allows many Capricorns to earn extra income from a favourite hobby. Work first — play later is the Capricorn philosophy but too much work and not enough play can be bad for you. You must strive to maintain a fair balance between your social and pleasurable pursuits and your regular responsibilities and commitments.

Sometimes you can neglect the lighter side of life and the company of friends, through becoming too absorbed in your latest project. Although you are not frivolous, you, more than most, need at least one close friend. Someone who understands you and is happy to share your triumphs and also sympathise if ever your plans fail. You are more of a mixer and a party-goer than is commonly thought, but prefer to stay in the background or on the fringe of the crowd unless you are called upon to entertain or take an active part. Parties and social gatherings are always a testing time for your figure because apart from your genuine liking for good food, you can be surprisingly vulnerable to over-eating if you are faced with a generous display of tempting dishes which include those you have always considered your favourites.

Your diet intentions can also be threatened when you go on holiday because this is one time you are ready to throw caution to the wind and seek adventure — looking for exciting places to explore. Even if you want to be a stick-in-the-mud in your food tastes you can come unstuck because exotic places often have equally exotic menus, so special thought must be given to the fattening implications of your order. Count the calories as well as the cost.

A gift that most Capricorns possess is an uncanny sense of timing which gives you a head start in games or pastimes which depend on team-work and precision, such as football, netball, rugby and hockey. You, better than most, understand about sticking to the rules, so will find it fairly easy to stick to your diet plan until you achieve your perfect weight. Sentence yourself to a lifetime of being slim, healthy and happy — knowing that you have earned your new, more attractive image.

AQUARIUS

January 20 — February 18

Ruled by two planets, Uranus the planet of change and Saturn the planet of structure, Aquarius is the "fixed" Air sign, suggesting that although Aquarians have an airy restlessness, they also seek stability. However, in common with Gemini and Libra, the other two Air signs, Aquarians need the freedom to circulate and to communicate their thoughts and ideas. Aquarius, which is the eleventh sign of the zodiac, is symbolised by The Water Bearer, representing Man carrying knowledge - this is why Aquarius is considered to be the sign of Humanity. Many Aquarians possess a strong social conscience; it is by making a positive contribution to their community that they find their true purpose.

YOUR SLIMMING CHARACTER

There are so many contradictions in your nature that others may be forgiven if they find it hard to understand you. Even the two planets which rule your sign are diverse in nature, as Uranus is a planet connected with change, originality and freedom, while Saturn is associated with limitation, patience and learning life's lessons the hard way. This curious combination you possess of mixed planetary strengths can now be used in your favour, because they are precisely the qualities you need to make a successful slimmer. Not only are you independent enough to refuse to stay, like a prisoner, bound to your fat, you are realistic enough to appreciate the sense of an organised diet-plan created with your personality in mind.

It's likely that you had a contrary streak in your nature from the time you were a child, because, as an Aquarian, you are a free spirit who resists doing what others want you to do — unless, of course, it's the same as you want. No doubt others view you as one of those people who sets their own rules and makes their own choices. You are now presented with the sort of choice which is easy for you to make since it gives you the chance to break free from the habits that tie you to old eating patterns. You can look forward to liberating the inner you, the one that is slim and dynamic. From the moment you make your mind up to tackle your weight problem, you are already well on the way to wearing a smaller size in clothes. Because once you arrive at a decision, you usually pursue it with tremendous energy and conviction.

YOUR SLIMMING WEAKNESSES

One of your greatest slimming weaknesses is your tendency to "make do" with food that's instantly available. In your book eating means refuelling and is a necessity rather than a grand passion. This means you grab a quick sandwich or eat up yesterday's left-overs, whatever they may be, when hungry, because whatever's going will serve the purpose of filling you up. The next time you feel like tucking into the remains of last night's sweet and sour, or apple tart, remember that you could soon be wearing the excess calories you're consuming. Instant food may temporarily satisfy your stomach, but it doesn't take long for your body's computer to do its sums and calculate whether its latest input contains sufficient nutrients and vitamins. If it doesn't, beware! Before you know it, that empty feeling will hit you again and both your appetite and waistline will grow larger and larger.

> **LOSE TO RAISE FUNDS**
> *Yours is the sign considered to be the most socially conscious of the zodiac, so why not organise a sponsored slim? While you're shedding pounds, which you're better off without anyway, you will have the extra pleasure of knowing you're raising money for the fight against hunger and poverty in the third world.*

As organising tomorrow and the future is important to you, you must avoid falling into another Aquarian classic slimming trap — rushing into the nearest food store to buy an essential item, such as milk or bread, and staggering out pounds lighter in cash but laden down with a huge box containing an assortment of biscuits, crisps, nuts, pies and other instantly edible foods which encourage you to gain those unsightly pounds you can do without. Stay away from the shops unless you are stocking up on essentials — and then stick to a carefully prepared list, which should be compiled after you've eaten and before the next meal becomes the uppermost thing on your mind.

Yet another of your slimming obstacles is something you were born with — that Uranian energy within which stirs you up every now and again and urges you to experiment and rebel against rules and regulations. Guard against varying your Astrodiet, which been carefully balanced, just for the buzz of being different. Following a recipe closely is not really your style, so whether or not the results are mouth watering or are delegated to the dog to eat, you can claim that every dish you concoct is an exclusive. Try to curb that adventurous streak a little and stay safely within the range of the suggested foods and portions in your Astrodiet. This is the only certain way to achieve your required weight loss, without any set-backs. By way of compensation, start planning to ring the changes with your wardrobe to suit the reduced you that's on the way.

YOUR SLIMMING STRENGTHS

You eat to live, rather than live to eat, which makes you an ideal candidate for a slimming diet. Here lies one of your greatest weapons in your fight against flab, as it stops food crowding your thoughts and constantly stimulating your appetite. As a busy Aquarian, you have plenty of interests other than your stomach. There are always a multitude of things to do and people to see. You will also appreciate the merits of a diet plan that makes your life flow more smoothly and the knowledge that this new eating plan will work for you without the hassle of wondering what to buy for the next meal — even if you're one of the packed-lunch brigade or fit in meals whenever possible according to your schedule. You can now eat at home and away without worrying

HIT THAT HABIT
Although you're interested in new ideas, you can sometimes be bound by old habits when it comes to your choice of food. On no account should you eat the same old vegetables all your life. As your Astrodiet lasts for seven days, why not eat a different vegetable on each one of them? Make a pact with yourself to experiment while slimming and look around for new tastes and shapes.

that your figure will suffer as a consequence.

You are honest with yourself, another of your great slimming strengths. You are prepared to accept the consequences of your own actions. Whenever your tape measure tells you that your current dimensions are "stretching" it a bit, or your weight is not to your liking or your doctor's, you don't blame it on depression or bad luck. This willingness to take responsibility for your life — and what you eat — is vital for any slimming regime to work and will save you from repeating any mistakes. Not only can you analyse the effects others have on your eating patterns but you can also pinpoint the type of situation which is bad for your figure.

Another plus factor, which will help you in your efforts to lose weight is the fact that you are your own person and not likely to be influenced by kindly, or, come to that, scathing comments on how you look. The decision to take positive action about losing weight is one you will make by yourself, for yourself — and once you do so, little will stand in your way. You need to be convinced that a new idea will work before you'll dive in at the deep end, but once you are impressed that it has a fair chance of success, you give it your best shot and need pretty powerful reasons to alter course. Aquarius is, after all, one of the three "fixed" signs, so there is a fixed, stubborn side to your nature, which will enable you to carry on dieting and exercising until you have arrived at exactly the shape and size you've set your heart on.

FREE TO CHOOSE

You need freedom to do your own thing, so your Astrodiet will suit you. As you are allowed to eat more food on some days than others you can swap the whole day's diet plan around if the pattern doesn't match your appetite. The smaller amounts allotted to weekdays allow you to indulge yourself a little at weekends or on special occasions, without worrying.

If you're a true blue Aquarian, you know your own worth and are also quick to weigh up others. You rarely undersell yourself. Whether you're negotiating money, love or chores, you know you deserve the best. This sense of self-worth can be the spur you need whenever you are tempted to break your sensible, new eating patterns for a quick but forbidden bite. Bear in mind that the outer you will become more like the inner you every day of your diet — slimmer, fitter and more attractive, inch by inch and pound by pound. Fortunately, you are ready to wait for what you want.

Your outlook is broad, unprejudiced and receptive to new thoughts and ideas. Being fair-minded and tolerant, you give others the chance to have their say, especially as you have strong views of your own which make you ready to fight for any cause in which you believe. Equality is a key word in the Aquarian vocabulary and so you consider slimming and keeping fit as important for men as it is for women. The right that everyone has to be proud of their body and to feel good about themselves is a wonderful cause for you to support now — and this book will help you to pursue it.

YOU AND YOUR BODY

There are so many thoughts buzzing around in your brain that you sometimes completely fail to listen to what your body's telling you. Do you find yourself putting off vital health and dental appointments because you're too busy in other directions? There's no point in fooling yourself, the truth is that you can't put off until tomorrow the sensible eating that must be done today. Your tendency to live in your head can be a contributory cause to problems that arise in your general well-being and a real threat to your hopes of becoming slim and fit unless you get to grips with it.

You, more than most, need to cultivate good habits relating to your health. Dieting needs to become part of your way of life, so that your body is always well-stocked with the essential vitamins and minerals that keep you charged with energy and glowing with health. The circulation and the ankles and calves are the parts of the body particularly associated with Aquarius — a sure indication that you should take special care of your legs and

SALAD CRAZE
Are all your salads the same? One lettuce leaf, two slices of cucumber and a half of tomato? Then it's definitely time for a change! Mix a whole new range of tastes and try a new dressing too, you could even make your own from vinegar and lemon juice with fresh herbs. You could also use cold pasta as the basis for a main course salad — try it with just a little cubed ham or grated cheese.

guard against such weight-related conditions as varicose veins. Skipping, jogging and aerobic exercises are representative of the sort of movements that can keep you in shape. Challenge your body with progressive exercise, rather than throwing yourself into a vigorous work out from day one. Exercise every day — this can be a brisk ten minute walk, a stint of gardening or some energetic housework, gradually building up to longer periods. Not only will daily exercise speed up your metabolism, you'll find your surplus weight will drop away as if by magic. The fact is that a once-a-week work-out has little effect on your regular weight.

In common with Gemini and Libra, the other two Air signs, you benefit from plenty of fresh air, whatever the weather, so don't forget to include plenty of outdoor activities in your programme.

YOU AND YOUR EMOTIONS

You look for a friend first, a lover second, because friendship is everything to you. You hate to lose a single pal, so are the world's worst at closing the door on a broken romance. Your philosophy is that a relationship doesn't end, it merely changes. Luckily for you, your appetite is rarely influenced by the state of your love life and whether you are giddy with excitement about a brand new passion, comfortably "settled down" or still looking, you munch food steadily through the sort of emotional dramas that knock other people's diet intentions for six. This is because you refuse to be a slave to your passions and only alter your eating patterns when it suits you to do so.

HEAD FOR HERBS
There's no need to always be a milk and sugar merchant (both add extra calories to drinks) where tea and coffee are concerned. Treat yourself to a selection of herbal teas — jasmine and peppermint are particularly refreshing. If you hanker for your old ways, compromise with black coffee or tea with lemon and you will never look back.

Many Aquarians marry young — usually before they become set in their ways. It can be hard for you to commit yourself again if your first attempts at finding wedded bliss fail. Subconsciously or not, you tend to search for an exact clone of your first love and it takes some Aquarians most of their lives to wake up to the fact that they will either have to remarry the same person or accept a different model. Ideally your partner must be as unpredictable as you —

sensible one minute, zany the next. They must also be intelligent without being a know-all. You can't stand pompous people. Above all, they must be self-sufficient because you soon shy away from anyone who is over-demanding as you dislike being pinned down or too committed. Even so, a commitment is called for now if you are to achieve the size and weight you desire.

You respond positively to those born under the other Air signs — Geminis, Librans and fellow Aquarians. This mix often works extremely well in a long-term relationship because it is a marriage of the minds. Not only do you speak the same language, there will always be plenty to talk about. You know how to handle each other and respect each other's right to space and freedom, which means you will be happy socialising apart as well as together with an Airy partner. If you start slimming with an Air person, expect to share lots of laughs as well as a wealth of interesting thoughts and ideas.

One thing you share with an Earth person — a Taurus, Virgo or Capricorn — is the ability to be rational. A relationship with a member of any of these signs starts off on a fairly realistic basis, so you could go far together, providing there are enough other things in common. An Earth partner will provide the back-up you need for your slimming regime, especially when you are going through one of your highly pressurised periods. At the same time, you can draw them out of themselves and help them to break down those reserves that Earth people tend to have, which can deprive them of the fun and lighter side of life. You can also encourage your Earth companions to think positively about the joy of being slim.

Fire people know how to excite you — Aries, Leos and Sagittarius are all very compatible with your sign. They, like you, enjoy social inter-action and new challenges. In a romantic relationship, there will be plenty of sparkle at first, but you will have to work at it to keep the love light burning brightly, as their enthusiasm to race ahead all the time could bring out the most stubborn side of your personality. You can count on the Fire members of your household to rally round when you announce that you intend to begin a new slimming diet. And, unless they are very thin, expect them to want to join in and show you how it is done. Let them!

It is a curious fact, that although a relationship with one of the Water people, a Cancer, Scorpio or Pisces, is never without its share of problems, you are irresistibly drawn to these signs and may therefore be married to, or have a Water person as one of your closest friends. Their uncanny intuition and sensitive feelings intrigue you and their ability to sense the mood of the moment and know when you are upset or overwrought never fails to astonish you. You both love and hate the caring a Water partner can give you as your basic urge to move unfettered by restrictions is threatened by a clinging Water-vine whose natural instinct is to belong to and hang on. Nevertheless, you could be pleasantly surprised if you enlist their help as a slimming supporter. You'll receive bags of encouragement, plus welcome assistance with shopping and meal preparation. You'll also be the recipient of well-meaning but unwanted advice — and sympathy which you'll loathe. If you decide to diet independently, watch out for sabotage as Water people resent feeling unneeded.

YOUR CREATIVE ENERGIES

There's nothing you like more than a brain teaser. You get a kick out of resolving problems. There's also a competitive edge to your personality, so you seek stimulus and challenge in your leisure activities. Check out the next suitable date on your personal Astrochart for beginning your diet and it won't be long before you can tell your friends and family that once again, you came up with the winning solution. You will derive an extra thrill out of proving to yourself that you found a way to do something positive to overcome your weight problem.

Next time you pass the first-aid person, the school crossing officer or the assistant in the Oxfam shop, stop and take a second look. Do they seem familiar? Chances are they're fellow Aquarians. Many Aquarians enjoy spending some of their leisure time in work that will help others, and it's likely that you have at least one spare-time activity that could be useful to the community.. (A sponsored slim is right up your street — you lose pounds to raise pounds — for your favourite charity.)

However, as the most group-conscious sign of the zodiac, social eating can pose a problem. Be especially aware of the impact the typical fare served up at a barbecue or garden party has on your midriff and pack your diet meal into your picnic basket so you can stay figure-conscious while you're eating out of doors. You enjoy the security of having a large circle of friends because they can rescue you when you fall into one of your regular spells of deep loneliness, which although rarely lasting for long, represent one of the most stressful times for your figure. Follow as many of your creative interests as possible in group situations or with at least one other person. As you rarely allow sentiment to sway your judgement, others look your way when they want a straight answer to a question, knowing that they will receive unbiased and well-considered advice. It is easy for you to spell out the obvious answer to a heavyweight friend who's worried about increasing girth, but you can be strangely resistant to taking advice yourself, unless you have asked for it especially.

You are fascinated by such things as space travel and laser beams and are not afraid of using computers and electronic gadgets in both your work and play. Once you involve yourself in a hobby, you tend to stick with it until the day that

CONSUMER NEWS
Be smart and arrange to eat with a fellow Aquarian or a Gemini or a Libra an your Danger days, because you'll be so busy exchanging stimulating ideas, news, views and information that you'll have little time left to nibble or even to contemplate the contents of your fridge.

something more interesting comes along. This tenacity in your character will allow you to give a new diet routine enough time to succeed. Being able to experiment and stamp your own individuality on your work is important to you, so projects which allow you to add your personal touch to them such as model making, specialist cooking and astrology often appeal to you. And as you have a practical slant, you are likely to be adept at many different handicrafts. Like the Water Bearer that symbolises your sign, you like being near the water and may therefore find boating, rowing, canoeing or sailing the ideal ways for you to spend a vacation. You are ready to "rough it" a little in order to go somewhere unusual or unconventional, providing it allows you to be with other people. An off-beat, action- packed holiday is far more to your taste than attempting to relax by being idle and less likely to tempt you to nibble away your boredom.

Your scales are likely to be an update on everyone else's, not to mention your can-opener and toothbrush. Because of all the twelve signs of the zodiac yours is the most inventive and eager to try anything new or different — like a slimming plan based on the stars. Others may regard you as unpredictable. Be glad that you are because that's what makes you so very special. Your free-thinking attitudes and your refusal to be type-cast, makes slimming so right for you — a progressive and exciting Aquarian.

PISCES

February 19 — March 19

PISCES, the sign of the Fish, which is the twelfth and last sign of the zodiac, is symbolised by two fish, tied by a cord but swimming in opposite directions, representing the duality that's at the heart of every Pisces. This dual theme is emphasised by the fact that two planets, Jupiter and Neptune, co-rule Pisces. As Jupiter governs expansion and opportunity and Neptune governs dreams and ideals, Pisces are usually very intuitive and able to form judgements by using their impressions and feelings. Associated with the element of Water, Pisces is also considered to be the most sensitive sign of the zodiac.

YOUR SLIMMING CHARACTER

You are the dreamer of the zodiac. As a child you may have lived in a world of fantasy and played many games of make-believe. Your inner conflicts often begin when the time comes to examine your dreams and be honest about which can be realised and which are pie in the sky. This book is especially valuable to you because it makes it possible for at least one of your most important dreams to come true — the dream all Pisces possess, to be slim, graceful and more attractive.

The two fish, which symbolise your sign, are usually depicted pointing away from each other, suggesting that Pisces have dual desires. If you reflect on your life you will probably agree that you often find yourself having to choose between two options, when you must decide whether to swim upstream or downstream. The fact that you're reading this book indicates that you are well aware of the right choice to make at the moment, where your overweight problem is concerned. Apart from the fact that you know too much fat is bad for your health, your appearance matters to you a great deal. Not only has your Astrodiet been carefully planned — but your Astrochart gives the exact date to begin. So what are you waiting for? Brace yourself and take the plunge — it will be a choice you'll never regret!

YOUR SLIMMING WEAKNESSES

Your greatest slimming weakness is procrastination. You don't necessarily put things off because you're lazy — but because you're afraid of failure. In fact fear of the unknown causes many Pisces to sentence themselves to a lifetime of suffering, in the mistaken belief that "the devil they know" is better than taking a chance. The wish to be slimmer and a size or two smaller may have been with you for a long time. You could have even been severely depressed about your weight problem, but instead of taking remedial action, may have pretended to your friends and colleagues that you liked being plump, rounded and cuddly, or claimed that fat people are jolly. But in your heart of hearts you know that something must be done to free yourself of those unwanted inches. Unfortunately you are rarely motivated to make a change until you feel secure in the knowledge that success is guaranteed. The results that will soon be apparent from even one week on your diet will provide you with all the reassurance you need. Expect to enjoy a steady weight loss and a general boost in your energy levels and sense of well-being.

FOOD FOR THE SOUL
Music is important to you, so the next time you feel tempted to raid your refrigerator for a slice of your favourite quiche or a crafty portion of cheese and biscuits, first try sitting down and playing or listening to your favourite selection of Mozart or McCartney. The chances are that filling your senses with melodious sounds will soon curb your appetite.

Your gentle Neptunian nature means that apart from finding it hard to be tough with others, you also you find it hard to be tough with yourself. As you know, the sight of a mouth-watering slice of pie winking at you from the open fridge is more than a poor Pisces can cope with. Store tasty leftovers in containers that are not the see-through type and you will find it easier to wait until your official meal time. Crash dieting is definitely not for you. The diet plan given in this book suits your need for a balanced and easy to follow eating pattern and will allow you to achieve your desired size without undue hardship.

Pisces is one of the three Water signs, the others being Cancer and Scorpio, so Water is your natural element. You must remember that what you drink is as important to your figure as what you eat. It is all too easy for you to get into the habit of sipping liquids without sparing a thought for their calorific content. You are far safer quenching your thirst with a cocktail of natural water and a splash of lemon, lime or orange, than pouring yourself out a double measure of a sugary soft drink which can jeopardise your best slimming efforts. In fact, drinks represent your secret enemies because they tend to pile on the pounds without filling your stomach.

Yours is an especially sensitive sign and it's also likely that you are very telepathic. You may often know who is on the other end of the phone before you have picked up the receiver, or what someone is going to say before they say it. You respond instinctively to others and possess a natural gift of being able to fathom out the mood of the moment and of knowing what others are thinking, sometimes acting like a sponge — you soak up impressions. This can be a weakness when it comes to shopping for and preparing food, because you could find yourself organising the meal that your partner or family is thinking about, whether or not it's bad news for your diet. You must constantly review your actions to ensure that what you are eating is uninfluenced by other people's thoughts, ideas, likes and dislikes.

You can be particularly influenced by the moods and dictates of others, so should make a point of surrounding yourself with positive, energetic people while you're slimming.

On no account should you dine with anyone who tries to dominate you, especially in regard to your choice of food. Those know-alls who think that

SNACK ATTACK

It's often the small snacks that are your downfall, so if you are conscious that you are inclined to nibble your way through the day, thereby eating too much, make it your business to set times and places where you ban yourself from eating food - even better if you can frequent those locations where it's inappropriate or anti-social to eat.

they know better than you about what's good for you could be a slimming obstacle, especially if they are unable to see why the four square meals a day, that they have eaten for years (all the way up to their present sixteen stone), is not, or is no longer, your style. In time, providing you follow your Astrodiet stringently, you will have them eating their words and, no doubt, envying you your slim shape and asking you the secret of your success!

YOUR SLIMMING STRENGTHS

Your sensitivity is one of your greatest assets in slimming. Not only are you sensitive to the messages your body sends to your brain, which provide a handy early-warning system for any trouble brewing, but you are also sensitive to the impact you make on others. Although at first you may be reluctant to admit to your friends that you're beginning a new diet regime (you do like to keep your little mysteries) the minute others comment favourably on your appearance will act like a spur to reinforce your efforts.

Pisces are sometimes accused of being wishy-washy or vague and indecisive but you know that this is not the case. You're far tougher than others may think, so even if trying to lose weight seems an uphill struggle at first, you possess the ability to get there in the end.

BE PREPARED

Have a grand sort-out of your wardrobe ready for your new, slimmer look. Make two separate piles, the clothes that will suit you later because they can be revamped or taken in — and those which are definitely designed for heavy-weights. Plan to take these to the charity shop or pass them on to a hard-up but tubby friend.

Receiving approval means a great deal to any Pisces, so you will probably go to tremendous lengths to win the respect and admiration of those you admire. This need to prove yourself can be a positive slimming advantage because knowing that you will soon be able to gaze into the mirror and congratulate yourself on the way you look, will do wonders for your self-confidence and help you to persevere with your diet.

Pisces are sometimes described as the poets of the zodiac as they are often blessed with vivid imagination and a wealth of inspired ideas. This fertile imagination is a definite point in your favour as a potential slimmer. Start imagining the attractive and fashionable clothes you will be able to wear once you have trimmed down to your desired shape and measurements.

In the end, you know that only you can control your eating

patterns. Fortunately you always feel more self-assured when Jupiter, one of your co-rulers, is in your sign or in a position in the heavens that is favourable for Pisces. You also stand to profit from the movement of Neptune, your other planetary ruler. The orbit of both these planets has been especially considered in the calculations of your Astrocharts. This will help you to organise your diary to allow for those days which could test your will-power and determination.

YOU AND YOUR BODY

You will have noticed that the planet Jupiter, associated with growth and expansion, is one of your co-rulers. Like Sagittarius, the other sign ruled by this benevolent planet, you can find yourself expanding literally as you grow older, with another millimetre round your waistline for every year of your age.

The parts of the body particularly associated with Pisces are the feet and the toes, so pamper your feet and give them all the loving care they deserve. Well-fitting shoes are an essential part of your wardrobe. Pinched toes soon make their uncomfortable presence felt and those Pisces smiles will soon fade if your feet are killing you. Your feet will also complain if the weight stacked up on top of them gets heavier and heavier and threatens to overload them. As you know, swelling ankles, corns, bunions and blisters, not

CREATURE COMFORTS
Sensitive and sometimes shy, Pisces people need to comfort themselves with activities that make the most of their natural imagination. When you are concentrating on painting a picture, learning a part in a play, or even writing a thrilling or romantic story, you are 'feeding' your creativity. Joining a class or an amateur dramatic society can often start a Pisces on a lifetime of rewarding experiences. Slimming becomes easier when you are happy.

to mention tender and burning heels and soles, are all part of the overweight problem. When you start to reduce your inches, don't be surprised if your toes curl up with pleasure, especially when you can treat yourself to shoes that are designed for a slim person rather than a fat one.

Like Cancers and Scorpios, the other two Water signs, your

weight tends to fluctuate according to your moods, so resist any temptation you may have to jump onto your bathroom scales every day. You'll obtain a more accurate picture of your progress by weighing in once a week at a regular time. It is the steady, constant effort invested in a diet plan that brings appreciable results.

Exercise routines that are enjoyable are a must for you because you can quickly become discouraged if slimming means suffering. Music is particularly important to a Pisces and helps take you out of yourself, so it provides you with an easy way of learning to relax and throw off the tensions of the day. Many Pisces love to dance but whether or not you're a Fred Astaire or Ginger Rogers doesn't really matter, because exercising to rhythm is a fun and effective way of shaping up and quickly shedding those extra pounds.

Pisces was considered by the ancient astrologers to be the sign of "one's own undoing" because of the idea that many Pisces fail to take what they want from life, or lack appreciation of what they already have — that is until it's gone. Learning to live in the now is one of your lessons in life. Instead of reminiscing about how slim you were once or speculating on how slim you might have been "if only", decide that your body is going to look the way you want it to look, going in and out in the right places and equally attractive from all angles. Forget about the chances you didn't take to slim. As from today, use the power of positive thought and refuse to be a wobbling example of the power of food. Also avoid dwelling for too long on the future — you can be assured that you will be rightfully proud of your appearance by the time it arrives.

JUST IMAGINE

You're an adventurous eater, so use your vivid imagination to make every single meal a brand new experience. Sprinkle ginger or cinnamon on fruit, add black peppercorns to fish, a dash of chili to sausages or meat, oregano on tomatoes or cheese and marjoram to pasta.

YOU AND YOUR EMOTIONS

Flirting and falling in love works miracles for your figure. The excitement, the sheer pleasure, the teasing, the chase and being close to someone special makes any thoughts of over-eating fly out of the window. Yours is a romantic sign and you love to be in love. Some Pisces spend an entire lifetime pining for the love that once was or the love that they long for but has never been. When you give your heart, you give it completely and often paint a glowing picture in your mind's eye of the one you have chosen, refusing to see their failings. You are a perfectionist, but when your heart is involved, you tend not to see people as they really are. Instead, you see them as you would like them to be. Even so, you can be too exacting and too critical of what life has to offer you, so guard against any inclination to turn to food and drink for comfort if the person you have devoted yourself to fails to come up to your expectations.

You offer sympathy and caring and are ready to make sacrifices for those who matter to you, such as your spouse or your family. Ideally you need a mate who is protective and supportive, who is also understanding and practical enough to prop you up in times of crisis. Your feelings run deep and your passions are strong, so you can be easily hurt, which means it's important for you to be especially discerning before allowing yourself to become emotionally involved in a relationship.

An interesting facet of your personality is the way you will listen to the tragedies of the world and accept them in a compassionate but philosophical fashion but find it hard to deal with the slightest emotional upset when it's one of your own, particularly if you fall in love with someone who doesn't reciprocate.

Your figure usually reflects the exact state of your romantic situation fairly accurately; your weight tends to monitor how much, or how little, love you are currently receiving.

If there are Fire signs in your family or circle of friends, you will already be well aware that they tackle life in a very different way to you. They take the bold, direct approach and are often extremely assertive, while your way is subtle and gently persuasive. When it comes to slimming with a Fire person you could just "pip them to the post" and succeed where they fail. This is because impatience is a common failing in the Fire personalities, who could abandon their diet plans when they discover that as fat cells burn less energy than muscles, they can only be reduced by establishing new, long-term eating health habits.

Gemini, Libra and Aquarius, the Air people, can also present a challenge to you, but not as much challenge as you do to them. Your ultra-sensitivity, which makes you easily hurt, and your ability to be inscrutable, so that no-one knows what you're planning, will both bother and bewilder curious Air signs. An Air person likes to rationalise thoughts, feelings and actions and bring them out into the open, so is unlikely to understand how you manage, without asking a single question, to make so many accurate assessments. Together you make a fairly restless combination, who will achieve most when you join up to work towards a mutual goal — so slimming together makes sense. Unless they have a common aim a Pisces and an Air person become absorbed in interests which cause them to drift apart, never really learning to understand what makes each other tick.

A partner born under one of the Earth signs, Taurus, Virgo or Capricorn, will provide the stability and solid support you need and help you to identify and realise your main aims in life. You are naturally sympathetic to each other, so this relationship should work well and also prove beneficial for weight-watching. Your perception will tell you the moment your Earth partner or friend is in danger of floundering, which means you have the chance gently to tease them out of breaking their diet. They can help you reorganise your larder, refrigerator or freezer, so you know exactly what's in stock or what to put on your shopping list.

Living with a fellow Water sprite — Pisces, Cancer or Scorpio — should prove mutually gratifying, as you offer comfort and emotional reinforcement for each other. There is usually a quiet, relaxed empathy between those born under the Water signs, which provides a sound basis for a long-term partnership. The biggest problem you must contend with, if you intend to diet along with another Water person, is your extreme receptivity to each other's moods. Both of you are inclined to be reactive and can, therefore, threaten each other's good diet resolutions, if either is having a down day. Your Astrochart will help you to overcome this hurdle as you will know ahead when to be especially diet-conscious.

YOUR CREATIVE ENERGIES

Many Pisces are blessed with great inspiration, which adds a special quality to their work, so it follows that Pisces men and women swell the ranks of the artists, poets, actors and musicians of society. Apart from these obvious artistic pursuits, there are many other ways that you express your creativity — through gardening, decorating, making lace, knitting, pottery, wood carving — the urge to create is strong in you and developing this creative side of your personality is a vital step towards your finding inner peace and fulfilment. That ability you have of losing yourself in whatever occupies your thoughts is another reason to regard your creative hobbies as important. You are not likely to nibble while creating a work of art — but you might do so while watching someone else's masterpiece on T.V.

You need plenty of music in your life because listening to music uplifts your spirits and puts you in a good frame of mind. The same applies if you are one of those gifted Pisces who plays a musical instrument, such as a keyboard, violin or guitar.

Your artistic efforts, whether of the practical or the fun kind, allow you to express your intense inner feelings in a positive and enjoyable way. Overeating and other indulgences, such as excessive smoking or drinking alcohol, are usually a form of escapism, so the key to maintaining a constant weight and a well body is to create a happy and interesting life for yourself.

GETTING STEAMED UP
Steaming is a super way to cook vegetables. And beneficial to your health as it doesn't boil away essential vitamins and mineral salts. Although steaming takes about the same time as boiling, you can put more than one vegetable in together without them fighting each other by spoiling each other's colour or flavour. Test for bite and don't overcook - they are tastiest when still on the crisp side.

Although you, more than most, need periods to be on your own, to repair the damage that the frantic world does to your nerves, you should guard against becoming too much of a loner or a stop-at-home. It's especially beneficial for you to join in group activities. A keep-fit class would be especially good or, as befits your natural sense of rhythm, a dancing class. You also often do well in sports and activities that depend on balance such as skiing, skating, yoga and water sports.

You cannot cope with discord so need to plan your off-duty moments carefully, especially your holidays. Look for places which offer peace, tranquillity and beauty when you next plan to take a vacation or a mini-break, as these are ideal for your dreamy Pisces soul. Finding yourself in uncomfortable accommodation or ugly surroundings is something you need to avoid at all costs. Trust your intuition if uncertain of where to go as it rarely lets you down. Your inner voice has also given you a clear message about your weight — it has guided you to this book, so pay attention and consult your Astrochart to discover the day to begin your diet,

the diet which is about to change your life and help you to make
your dreams come true.

THE ASTRODIETS

The following diet plans will help you to lose weight safely and are designed especially with your astrological type in mind. They will also assist in establishing a healthy pattern of eating for the future. You will find it easy to stay slim once you have achieved your ideal weight if you continue to follow the guidelines given. In the introduction to each diet are instructions for repeating it, for more effective results, and if you have a lot of weight to lose, you will have to do this. Whether you are folowing a Fire, Earth, Air or Water diet, use it as the basis for your eating patterns for the rest of your life. Your Astrodiet will allow you to eat well and wisely, so that you need never look back or become overweight again.

THE DIET FOR FIRE SIGNS
(Aries, Leo, Sagittarius)

This diet allows you six meals a day, and yet will result in a speedy weight loss. Surprisingly, perhaps, eating more often can be a very effective way to slim - because it keeps your metabolism "revved up" and stops your system from feeling and reacting as if it were being starved of supplies. Not only are the results quick - the meals on the diet are also quick and easy to prepare. Once the week is up, you should return to normal eating, but of course you will have to watch your intake if your weight is not to shoot up again. So don't go back to bad old habits - use what you learn on this diet as a guide to healthy eating for the future. On occasion, you can repeat any two days of the diet to offset a heavier-eating event — like Christmas — and help to keep your weight where you want it to be. However,do not repeat the diet in its entirety more frequently than once in every six weeks.
YOU MUST DRINK 6-8 GLASSES OF WATER EVERY DAY.
NOTE: It is always wise to check with your GP before starting on any diet particularly if you have a health problem.

DAY ONE

Meal 1:
1 Weetabix with 1 banana, sliced and 4 fl. oz./l25ml semi-skimmed milk; tea or coffee, black or with semi-skimmed milk, *no sugar* (you may use a sweetener)
Meal 2:
3 oz./75g grapes
Meal 3:
4 oz./l00g smoked mackerel, 1 tomato, 5oz. /125g.pot of diet coleslaw, 1 slice wholemeal bread
Meal 4:
8 oz./250g any combination of raw salad vegetables (choose from beetroot, cabbage, cauliflower, celery, chicory, cucumber, peppers, radishes, spring onions)*
Meal 5:
2 low-fat sausages, grilled and served with 4 oz./l00g canned chopped tomatoes and 2 oz./50g brown rice, boiled
Meal 6:
1 apple
In addition: 2 cups tea or coffee, black or with semi-skimmed milk, *no sugar* (you may use a sweetener)

DAY TWO

Meal 1:
1 oz./25g bran cereal with 1/2oz./12g sultanas and 4 fl. oz./125 ml semi-skimmed milk; tea or coffee, black or with semi-skimmed milk, *no sugar* (you may use a sweetener)
Meal 2:
2 satsumas
Meal 3:
2-slice wholemeal sandwich of 1 teaspoon low-fat spread mixed with 2 oz./50g Edam cheese, grated, and 1 tablespoon tomato ketchup plus cucumber slices.
Meal 4:
As Day One
Meal 5:
2 low-fat beefburgers, grilled with 1 tomato, halved and grilled and 5 oz./125g baked beans in tomato sauce
Meal 6:
1 pear
In addition: 2 cups tea or coffee, black or with semi-skimmed milk, *no sugar* (you may use a sweetener)

DAY THREE

Meal 1:
1 Weetabix with 1 apple, chopped, and 4 fl. oz./125ml semi-skimmed milk; tea or coffee, black or with semi-skimmed milk, *no sugar* (you may use a sweetener)

Meal 2:
2 oz./50g cottage cheese and 2 crispbreads

Meal 3:
$3^1/2$ oz./90g tuna, canned in brine, with 2 oz./50g sweetcorn, drained, 4 oz./l00g cold, cooked green beans, 2 oz./50g canned red kidney beans, and 2 tablespoons/30ml low-calorie vinaigrette dressing

Meal 4:
as Day One

Meal 5:
4 oz./l00g roast or baked chicken, NO SKIN, with a 4 oz./l00g jacket-baked potato, dressed with 1 tablespoon/15ml low-fat natural yoghurt plus 4 oz./l00g any green vegetable, steamed

Meal 6:
2 satsumas.

In addition: 2 cups tea or coffee, black or with semi-skimmed milk, *no sugar* (you may use a sweetener).

DAY FOUR

Meal 1:
1 oz./25g bran cereal with half oz./12g dried apricots, chopped, and 4 fl. oz./125ml semi-skimmed milk; tea or coffee, black or with semi-skimmed milk, *no sugar* (you may use a sweetener)

Meal 2:
3 oz./75g grapes

Meal 3:
2-slice wholemeal sandwich of 1 hard-boiled egg, chopped and mixed with a punnet of mustard and cress and 1 tablespoon low-calorie salad cream

Meal 4:
as Day One

Meal 5:
6 oz./150g white fish, grilled and served with lemon and parsley, plus 4 oz./l00g potatoes, boiled and 2 oz./50g peas, boiled.

Meal 6:
3 slices of pineapple, fresh or tinned without sugar.

In addition: 2 cups tea or coffee, black or with semi-skimmed milk, *no sugar* (you may use a sweetener)

DAY FIVE

Meal 1:
1 Weetabix with 1 banana, sliced and 4 fl. oz./125ml semi-skimmed milk; tea or coffee, black or with semi-skimmed milk, *no sugar* (you may use a sweetener)
Meal 2:
2 crispbreads spread with 1 teaspoon of Marmite and topped with 1 tomato, halved
Meal 3:
2-slice wholemeal sandwich of 1 slice lean ham with 1 processed cheese slice and lettuce
Meal 4:
as Day One
Meal 5:
5 oz./125g jacket-baked potato, topped with 2 oz./50g cottage cheese and chives
Meal 6:
1 apple
In addition: 2 cups tea or coffee, black or with semi-skimmed milk, *no sugar* (you may use a sweetener)

DAY SIX

Meal 1:
1 egg, poached or boiled, and 1 slice wholemeal bread or toast with a scraping of low-fat spread; tea or coffee, black or with semi-skimmed milk, *no sugar* (you may use a sweetener)
Meal 2:
1 banana with 1 oz./25g chopped dates
Meal 3:
1 oz./25g cold cooked pasta with 2 oz./50g cottage cheese and 4 black olives, chopped in
Meal 4:
as Day One
Meal 5:
4 x 1 oz./25g slices lean ham wrapped around 4 sticks of pre-cooked broccoli topped with 2 processed cheese slices and browned under a hot grill, served with 2 oz./50g sweetcorn
Meal 6: 3 slices of pineapple, fresh or tinned without sugar
In addition: 2 cups tea or coffee, black or with semi-skimmed milk, no sugar (you may use a sweetener)

DAY SEVEN

Meal 1:
 1 rasher lean bacon, grilled with 1 tomato, halved and grilled
and 1 slice wholemeal toast; tea or coffee, black or with semi-
skimmed milk, no sugar (you may use a sweetener)
Meal 2:
 1 slice of wholemeal bread or toast spread with 1 teaspoon/5ml
honey
Meal 3:
 2 oz./50g prawns, mixed with 2 sticks celery, chopped, and a
half a small apple, chopped, and dressed with 1 teaspoon/5ml
low-calorie salad dressing and 1 teaspoon/5ml tomato ketchup
plus a dash of lemon juice, 1 slice wholemeal bread
Meal 4:
 as Day One
Meal 5:
4 oz./l00g liver, shredded and dry-fried with half a small onion,
chopped, 2 oz./50g mushrooms, sliced, and 1 tomato, skinned
and chopped, served with 2 oz./50g brown rice, boiled, and 4
oz./l00g spinach, steamed.
Meal 6:
 remaining half apple, chopped and served with 1 small orange,
segmented, 1 small banana, sliced and 2 oz./50g grapes
sprinkled with a little fresh orange juice
In addition: 2 cups tea or coffee, black or with semi-skimmed
milk, *no sugar* (you may use a sweetener)

NOTE: You must eat the full quantity of salad vegetables
each day. However, if you find it too much at a sitting, you
may instead add a little to other meal menus, or even snack
on salad as additional mini-meals.

THE DIET FOR EARTH SIGNS
(Taurus, Virgo, Capricorn)

This diet consists of three planned meals per day plus a treat. The diet is fairly strict and must be followed exactly, apart from the optional daily treat which can be exchanged for some fresh fruit if you prefer. You can follow this diet for one or two weeks at a time and repeat as often as two weeks in every six. You must, of course, eat sensibly for the rest of the time. It's important to weigh and measure portions carefully and avoid guesswork.

YOU MUST DRINK 6—8 GLASSES OF WATER EVERY DAY.

NOTE: It is always wise to check with your GP before starting any diet - particularly if you have a health problem.

EVERY DAY you're allowed half a pint/300 ml of skimmed milk - in addition to any milk listed on the diet — and unlimited tea or coffee, using milk from the allowance, but *no sugar* (you may use a sweetener). You are also allowed 1 slice of wholemeal bread in addition to any bread listed. Where no quantity is given for a vegetable, you may eat an unlimited amount.

DAY ONE
BREAKFAST:
half a grapefruit
1¹/₂oz./37g unsweetened bran or oat cereal
4 fl. oz./125ml skimmed milk
LIGHT MEAL:
2 oz./50g Edam cheese salad vegetables
1 granary roll
1 apple
MAIN MEAL:
3¹/₂oz./90g bacon steak, grilled with
1 pineapple ring and
half a tomato
YOUR TREAT:
1 doughnut

DAY TWO
BREAKFAST:
4 fl. oz./125 ml unsweetened orange juice
1 egg, poached, on 1 slice wholemeal toast
scraping of low-fat spread
LIGHT MEAL:
2 oz./50g beefburger, grilled
salad vegetables
1 pear
MAIN MEAL:
6 oz./175g cod fillet, grilled with a
scraping of low-fat spread
5 oz./125g potato, steamed or boiled
French beans
carrots
1 low-fat fruit yoghurt
YOUR TREAT:
a packet of crisps

DAY THREE
BREAKFAST:
4 fl. oz./125ml tomato juice
1 rasher lean back bacon, grilled
2 oz./50g mushrooms, simmered in stock
1 slice wholemeal toast
LIGHT MEAL:
3½oz./90g can tuna in brine
salad vegetables
1 orange
MAIN MEAL:
4 oz./100g liver, grilled
1½ oz./37g brown rice, boiled or steamed
spinach
carrots
8 oz./250g wedge of melon
YOUR TREAT:
2 oz./50g chocolate

DAY FOUR
BREAKFAST:
half a grapefruit
1½ oz./37g unsweetened bran or oat cereal
4 fl. oz./125ml skimmed milk
LIGHT MEAL:
2 oz./50g lean ham
salad vegetables
3 oz./75g grapes
MAIN MEAL:
5 oz./150g chicken joint, baked, NO SKIN
4 oz./100g jacket-baked potato, served with
1 tablespoon/15ml low-fat natural yoghurt
cauliflower
sweetcorn
strawberries, in natural juice
YOUR TREAT:
1 currant bun or scone with a scraping of low-fat spread

DAY FIVE
BREAKFAST:
4 fl. oz./125ml unsweetened orange juice
1 egg, boiled
1 slice wholemeal toast
scraping of low-fat spread
LIGHT MEAL:
4 oz./100g baked beans in tomato sauce on
1 slice wholemeal toast
1 orange
MAIN MEAL:
6 oz./175g plaice, grilled with a
scraping of low-fat spread
4 oz./l00g potato, steamed or boiled
celery hearts
carrots
pineapple slices, in natural juice
YOUR TREAT:
2 oz./50g sweets

DAY SIX
BREAKFAST:
2 fishcakes, grilled
2 tomatoes, grilled
LIGHT MEAL:
4 oz./lOOg cottage cheese
salad vegetables
1 apple
MAIN MEAL:
2 small lamb cutlets (maximum raw weight 4 oz./100g each),
grilled cauliflower
peas
carrots
8 oz./250g wedge of melon
YOUR TREAT:
2 oz./50g salted peanuts

DAY SEVEN

BREAKFAST:
2 eggs, scrambled with
1 tablespoon/15ml skimmed milk, and
scraping of low-fat spread
LIGHT MEAL:
salad vegetables ONLY
MAIN MEAL:
4 oz./100g lean roast beef in gravy
4 oz./100g roast potatoes - cut in large pieces
Brussels sprouts
parsnips
2 oz./50g vanilla ice cream
1 peach, fresh or tinned without sugar
YOUR TREAT:
2oz./50g peppermint creams

THE DIET FOR AIR SIGNS
(Aquarius, Gemini, Libra)

This is a do-it-yourself diet, so you may devise your own meals and snacks from the foods listed for each day - which have been balanced nutritionally and calorie counted, to ensure a healthy and effective weight loss. You may combine the foods in any way you wish, but you must only cook them as directed. For flavour, you may add seasonings, herbs or spices, clear stock, vinegar or lemon juice; and up to l tablespoon/15 ml of low-calorie salad dressing, tomato ketchup or brown sauce each day. You are also allowed one sweet or alcoholic treat daily. This is listed last, but you may have it at any time you wish, or you may substitute fresh fruit. Apart from these additions, do not eat anything other than the foods and beverages listed for each day - and do not omit any. (If there is an item which you are unable to tolerate, replace it with something from the same food group - i.e. replace protein with protein, carbohydrate with carbohydrate, etc - and of a similar calorie value.)
YOU MUST DRINK 6-8 GLASSES OF WATER EVERY DAY.

NOTE: It is always wise to check with your GP before starting any diet particularly if you have a health problem.

DAY ONE

2-4 cups of tea, with lemon or semi-skimmed milk, *no sugar* (you may use a sweetener)

2-4 cups of coffee, black or with semi-skimmed milk, *no sugar* (you may use a sweetener)

4 fl. oz./125 ml unsweetened orange or grapefruit juice

2 oz./50g unsweetened bran cereal

4 fl. oz./125 ml semi-skimmed milk

2 slices wholemeal bread or toast

1/2oz./12g low-fat spread

2 eggs (poached, boiled or cooked with low-fat spread - allowance above)

unlimited salad vegetables (choose from lettuce, cucumber, celery, peppers, tomatoes, beetroot, watercress, mustard and cress)

4 oz./100g chicken, NO SKIN (cooked any way except fried)

6 oz./150g potato, preferably with skin (steamed, baked or boiled)

6 oz./150g any green vegetables (steamed)

4 oz./100g carrots (steamed)

1 small pot low-fat natural yoghurt

1 pear

1 orange

TREAT:

4 fl. oz./125ml glass of any white wine

DAY TWO

2-4 cups of tea, with lemon or semi-skimmed milk, *no sugar* (you may use a sweetener)

2-4 cups of coffee, black or with semi-skimmed milk, *no sugar* (you may use a sweetener)

1 whole grapefruit

2 oz./50g muesli

4 fl. oz./125 ml semi-skimmed milk

2 slices wholemeal bread or toast

1/2oz./12g low-fat spread

4 oz./100g cottage cheese

unlimited salad vegetables (detailed on Day One)

6 oz./150g white fish (steamed, poached or baked)

6 oz./150g potato, preferably with skin (steamed, baked or boiled)

6 oz./150g any green vegetables (steamed)

2 oz./50g canned sweetcorn

half a melon

2-3 figs

TREAT:

1 Quaker Harvest Crunch or Harvest Chewy Bar, any flavour

DAY THREE

2-4 cups of tea, with lemon or semi-skimmed milk, *no sugar* (you
may use a sweetener)
2-4 cups of coffee, black or with semi-skimmed milk, *no sugar* (you
may use a sweetener)
1 whole orange
2 oz./50g unsweetened bran cereal
4 fl. oz./125ml semi-skimmed milk
2 slices wholemeal bread or toast
1/2oz./12g low-fat spread
4oz./100g tuna canned in brine
unlimited salad vegetables (detailed on Day One)
2oz./50g rice, preferably brown (boiled or steamed)
4oz./100g liver or kidneys
6 oz./150g any green vegetables (steamed)
3 oz./75g carrots (steamed)
2 oz./50g vanilla ice cream
4 oz./l00g raspberries, fresh, frozen or canned (without sugar)
1 pear
TREAT:
1 pub measure (50ml/1/3gill) Cinzano, Dubonnet or Martini

DAY FOUR

2-4 cups of tea, with lemon or semi-skimmed milk, NO SUGAR (you
may use a sweetener)
2-4 cups of coffee, black or with semi-skimmed milk, NO SUGAR
(you may use a sweetener)
4 fl. oz./125ml unsweetened orange or grapefruit juice
2 slices wholemeal bread or toast
1/2oz./12g low-fat spread
2 tablespoons/30ml honey
unlimited salad vegetables (detailed on Day One)
2 oz./50g pasta, preferably wholemeal
2 oz./50g Edam cheese
6 oz./150g tomatoes, fresh or canned
3 oz./75g lean ham
6 oz./150g any green vegetables (steamed)
1 apple
1 orange
1 oz./25g raisins
TREAT:
1 fun size Mars Bar or Milky Way

DAY FIVE

2-4 cups of tea, with lemon or semi-skimmed milk, *no sugar* (you may use a sweetener)
2-4 cups of coffee, black or with semi-skimmed milk, *no sugar* (you may use a sweetener)
1 whole grapefruit
2 oz./50g unsweetened bran cereal
4 fl. oz./125g semi-skimmed milk
2 slices wholemeal bread or toast
$1/2$ oz./12g low-fat spread
4 oz./l00g cottage cheese
unlimited salad vegetables (detailed on Day One)
2 oz./50g lean minced beef
2 oz./50g rice, preferably brown (steamed or boiled)
4 oz./l00g any green vegetables, steamed
2 oz./50g red kidney beans, canned
4 oz./l00g tomatoes, fresh or canned
4 oz./l00g onion (boiled or baked)
1 small pot low-fat fruit yoghurt
1 banana
$1/2$ melon
TREAT: 4 fl. oz./125ml glass any red wine

DAY SIX

2-4 cups of tea, with lemon or semi-skimmed milk, *no sugar* (you may use a sweetener)
2-4 cups of coffee, black or with semi-skimmed milk, *no sugar* (you may use a sweetener)
1 whole orange
2 oz./50g muesli
4 fl. oz./125ml semi-skimmed milk
2 slices wholemeal bread or toast
$1/2$oz./12g low-fat spread
4 oz./l00g prawns
unlimited salad vegetables (detailed on Day One)
4 oz/l00g chicken, NO SKIN (cooked any way except fried)
6 oz./150g potato, preferably with skin (steamed, baked or boiled)
6 oz./150g any green vegetables (steamed)
4 oz./l00g swede, turnip or parsnip (steamed)
4 oz./l00g grapes
1 peach, fresh or 6 oz./150g tinned without sugar
TREAT:
pub measure (25ml/$1/3$gill) any liqueur

DAY SEVEN

2-4 cups of tea, with lemon or semi-skimmed milk, *no sugar* (you
may use a sweetener)
2-4 cups of coffee, black or with semi-skimmed milk, *no sugar* (you
may use a sweetener)
4 fl. oz./125ml unsweetened orange or grapefruit juice
2 eggs (poached, boiled or cooked with low-fat spread - allowance
below)
1 slice wholemeal bread or toast
1/2 oz./12g low-fat spread
unlimited salad vegetables (detailed on Day One)
4 oz./l00g tuna, canned in brine
4 oz./l00g lean roast pork or beef, NO FAT
4 oz./l00g potato, preferably with skin (steamed, baked or boiled)
6 oz./150g any green vegetables (steamed)
6 oz./150g any root vegetables (steamed)
2 tablespoons/30ml fat-free gravy
1 apple
1 pear
1 orange.
TREAT: 1 Mr. Kipling French Fancy individual iced cake

THE DIET FOR WATER SIGNS
(Pisces, Cancer, Scorpio)

This is a pick-and-choose diet. Seven breakfasts, seven light meals and seven main meals are listed — and you can choose which you have when. And, in case there's a meal you don't like, you can miss any one light or main meal and repeat another. You may also repeat the same breakfast every day if you wish — unless it is a breakfast of an egg, which can be repeated only four times at the most in one week; but you may stick to just one or two favourite breakfasts if you prefer. Five of the light meals can be packed and carried, if you work away from home. To stay slim after your dieting week, you can repeat any of the meal combinations on up to four days a week, and eat normally — not over the top — on the other days. YOU MUST DRINK 6-8 GLASSES OF WATER EVERY DAY. NOTE: It is always wise to check with your GP before starting any diet - particularly if you have a health problem.

BREAKFASTS
half grapefruit
1 egg, boiled
3 crispbreads ½oz./12g low-fat spread
tea or coffee, black or with semi-skimmed milk, *no sugar* (you may use a sweetener)
••••••••••
4 fl. oz./125ml unsweetened orange juice
2 oz./50g any cereal, unsweetened
4 fl. oz./125ml semi-skimmed milk
tea or coffee, black or with semi-skimmed milk, *no sugar* (you may use a sweetener)
••••••••••
5 fl. oz./l50ml tomato juice
5 oz/125g baked beans in tomato sauce on
1 slice wholemeal toast
tea or coffee, black or with semi-skimmed milk, *no sugar* (you may use a sweetener)
••••••••••
4 fl. oz./125ml unsweetened grapefruit juice
2 fishcakes, grilled
1 tomato, grilled
tea or coffee, black or with semi-skimmed milk, *no sugar* (you may use a sweetener)
••••••••••
half a grapefruit
2 rashers lean bacon, grilled
2 oz./50g mushrooms, poached in water with a dash of Worcester sauce
tea or coffee, black or with semi-skimmed milk, *no sugar* (you may use a sweetener)
••••••••••
half a grapefruit
2 slices wholemeal bread or toast
½ oz./12g low-fat spread
2 teaspoons/l0ml jam, marmalade or honey
tea or coffee, black or with semi-skimmed milk, *no sugar* (you may use a sweetener)
••••••••••
1 whole orange
1 slice wholemeal bread, spread with

1 teaspoon/5ml Marmite, and topped with
2 tomatoes, halved
tea or coffee, black or with semi-skimmed milk, NO SUGAR
(you may use a sweetener)

LIGHT MEALS

4 oz./l00g cottage cheese OR 2 oz./50g Edam cheese
mixed salad vegetables of your choice
1 teaspoon/5 ml low-calorie salad dressing
1 slice wholemeal bread
scraping of low-fat spread
1 piece any fresh fruit up to 5 oz./125g weight
....
2 oz./50g prawns, dressed with
1 teaspoon/5ml low-calorie salad dressing PLUS
1 teaspoon/5ml tomato ketchup
mixed salad vegetables of your choice
1 slice wholemeal bread
scraping of low-fat spread
1 piece any fresh fruit up to 5 oz./125g in weight
....
2 oz./50g lean ham
2 oz./50g cottage cheese
2 tomatoes
1 slice wholemeal bread
scraping of low-fat spread
1 piece any fresh fruit up to 5 oz./125g in weight
....
3 1/2oz./90g tuna canned in brine
2 oz./50g chopped celery
1 oz./25g chopped onion
lettuce
1 teaspoon low-calorie salad dressing
1 slice wholemeal bread
scraping of low-fat spread
1 piece any fresh fruit up to 5 oz./125g in weight
....
1 egg, hard-boiled
half a punnet mustard and cress
1 teaspoon/5ml low-fat salad dressing
lettuce
1 slice wholemeal bread

scraping of low-fat spread
1 piece any fresh fruit up to 5 oz./125g in weight
···········
4 fish fingers, grilled
2 oz./50g peas, boiled
1 tomato, halved and grilled
mixed salad of any three fresh fruits, maximum weight 8 oz./250g
···········
2 oz./50g low-fat beefburger, fresh or frozen, grilled
5 oz./125g baked beans in tomato sauce
1 tomato, halved and grilled
mixed salad of any three fresh fruits, maximum weight 8 oz./250g

MAIN MEALS
3 1/2oz./90g gammon steak, topped with
1 slice pineapple, fresh or canned without sugar
half tomato
1 1/2oz./37g brown rice, boiled with
half a small onion, chopped
half a tomato, skinned and chopped, and
1 oz./25g mushrooms, chopped
1 oz./25g sweetcorn
6 oz./l50g cabbage, shredded and steamed with
1/4 green pepper, de-seeded and sliced in strips
2 oz./5Og vanilla ice cream
···········
3 oz./75g cold,cooked lean pork, cubed
1 1/2oz./37g dried apricots, chopped (soaked overnight in orange juice)
1 1/2oz/37g brown rice, boiled with
half a small onion, chopped
combined, and served on a bed of
6 oz./l50g spinach, steamed and shredded
1 low-fat fruit yoghurt
···········
6 oz./l50g breast of chicken, *no skin*, baked in foil spread with scraping of low-fat spread, with 1 teaspoon/5ml lemon juice, 1 crushed clove of garlic, and 1 tablespoon/l5ml fresh parsley, chopped finely
4 oz./l00g broccoli, steamed

2 oz./50g carrots, steamed
5 oz./125g jacket-baked potato, served with
1 tablespoon/15 ml low-fat natural yoghurt
2 oz./50g vanilla ice cream
•••••••••

1 bag frozen cod in butter or parsley sauce
5 oz./125g jacket-baked potato
6 oz./l50g sliced green beans, steamed
3 oz./75g swede, diced and steamed
1 low-fat fruit yoghurt
•••••••••

2 oz./50g lean minced beef, dry-fried with
4 oz./l00g canned chopped tomatoes with herbs
half a small onion, chopped, and served on
1¹/₂oz./37g wholemeal spaghetti, boiled
2 oz./50g peas, boiled
2 oz./50g vanilla ice cream
•••••••••

6 oz./l50g any white fish, steamed or baked with herbs of
choice
4 oz./l00g potatoes, steamed
4 oz./l00g sliced green beans, steamed
4 oz./l00g carrots, steamed
2 oz./50g vanilla ice cream
•••••••••

4 oz./l00g lean braising beef, cooked with water to cover, and
1 bay leaf
1 teaspoon/5ml tomato puree
4 oz./l00g carrots, sliced
4 oz./l00g potatoes, cut into chunks, and
1 small onion, sliced
6 oz./l50g leeks, steamed
1 low-fat fruit yoghurt

THE
ASTROCHARTS

ARIES

1990

1990	1	2	3	4	5	6	7	8	9	10	11	12	13	14	15	16	17	18	19	20	21	22	23	24	25	26	27	28	29	30	31
JAN																															
FEB																															
MAR																															
APR	✗	✗			✓	✗	✗	✗	✗	✗					✓					✓			✓	✓			✓		✗	✗	
MAY		✓									✓	✗								✓				✓		✗	✗		✓		
JUN		✗	✗				✗	✓			✓	✓									✓	✗	✗	✗		✓			✗	✗	
JUL	✗			✓		✓	✗	✗						✓	✓		✓	✓		✗	✗		✓	✗			✗	✗			
AUG	✓					✓	✓	✓		✓	✓		✗	✗		✗	✗		✗	✓			✓	✗			✗	✓			
SEP					✓			✓	✓			✓	✓	✗		✗	✗	✗	✗	✗			✗				✓			✓	✓
OCT					✓				✓														✓				✓	✗	✓		
NOV	✓					✗			✓							✓	✓		✓				✓					✗	✓		
DEC		✓		✗	✗	✓				✗						✓	✓	✗	✗										✓		✗

TAURUS

1990

1990	1	2	3	4	5	6	7	8	9	10	11	12	13	14	15	16	17	18	19	20	21	22	23	24	25	26	27	28	29	30	31
JAN																															
FEB																															
MAR																															
APR				✗	✗	✓	✓				✗	✗		✗		✓	✓		✗		✓	✓	✓	✓	✓	✓			✓	✓	
MAY	✗	✗	✓	✓		✓		✗	✗	✗																		✗	✗	✗	✓
JUN	✓									✓	✓								✓	✓		✓	✓	✓	✗	✗	✓	✓			
JUL		✗	✗			✗	✓	✓		✗						✓	✓					✗	✗	✓	✓	✗			✗	✗	✗
AUG						✗		✓	✓	✓			✓	✓				✗	✗	✗	✓	✓			✗	✗					
SEP		✗	✗			✓	✓		✓						✗	✗											✓	✓		✓	
OCT						✓	✓					✗	✗	✓			✓	✓						✓	✓	✓	✗		✓		
NOV		✓	✓				✗	✗	✗			✓			✗	✗	✗		✗	✓			✗	✗		✗				✗	
DEC	✓					✗	✗	✓			✗	✗	✗	✗				✓		✗	✗							✓			

1990

GEMINI — 1990

1990	1	2	3	4	5	6	7	8	9	10	11	12	13	14	15	16	17	18	19	20	21	22	23	24	25	26	27	28	29	30	31
JAN																															
FEB																															
MAR																															
APR		✓	✗	✗	✓	✓✗	✗			✓	✗	✗	✗	✗	✗✗					✓							✓	✓			
MAY	✗										✗	✗	✗	✗	✗	✓			✗			✓		✓	✓	✓	✓	✗			✗
JUN				✗	✗	✗	✗	✗		✓		✓	✗	✗				✓	✓		✓	✓	✓	✗	✗		✗	✗			
JUL						✓		✗		✓							✗	✓	✓	✓	✗	✗	✓								
AUG	✗				✗	✓		✗			✓	✓	✓		✓	✓	✗	✗	✗	✓	✓✗	✗		✗	✗		✗	✗✗	✗		
SEP			✓	✓✗	✗			✓	✓		✓	✓	✓		✓	✓		✓	✗	✓								✓		✓	
OCT	✓	✓✗		✓✗	✓							✗						✗	✗						✗					✗	✓
NOV	✓	✓			✓				✗		✗	✗	✓					✗	✗		✗	✗	✗	✗	✗			✓		✗	
DEC		✓✓	✓			✓		✗	✗	✓	✓				✗	✗				✓			✗	✗						✓	

CANCER

	1	2	3	4	5	6	7	8	9	10	11	12	13	14	15	16	17	18	19	20	21	22	23	24	25	26	27	28	29	30	31
JAN																															
FEB																															
MAR																															
APR	✗	✓	✓	✓	✗	✓	✗	✗	✗	✗	✓		✗	✗		✗	✗			✗	✗				✓	✓			✓	✓	
MAY			✓		✓			✓	✓	✓					✓												✓	✓			
JUN	✓	✗	✗	✗		✗	✗		✗	✗	✗						✗												✗	✗	
JUL	✗	✓	✓					✗					✓	✗	✗	✓				✓	✓		✓	✓			✗	✗		✓	
AUG			✗	✓	✓	✗	✗	✓	✓	✗	✗		✓	✓			✓	✓	✓	✗	✗	✓	✗	✗			✓			✗	
SEP	✗									✓	✓				✓								✓		✗	✗	✗	✗			
OCT		✓		✗			✓			✓					✓	✓	✗	✗		✗	✗			✗					✓		✗
NOV	✗	✓				✓		✓				✓	✗	✗			✓					✗						✗		✓	
DEC				✓	✓					✗	✗	✗		✓			✗	✗	✗						✗	✗		✓			✓

LEO

1990

1990	1	2	3	4	5	6	7	8	9	10	11	12	13	14	15	16 17	18	19	20	21	22	23	24	25	26	27	28	29	30	31
JAN																														
FEB																														
MAR																														
APR			X	✓	✓					✓	X	X	X		✓	X	X	X	X					X	X	X				
MAY		✓		X	X	X		X	X	X	✓					X X						X	✓					X	X	
JUN			✓			X	✓	✓	X	X	X	X	X				✓		X	✓		✓		✓	✓					
JUL						X	X		X	X	X	X					✓							X	X	X		X	X	X	X
AUG	✓	✓	X			✓		X	X		X	X		✓	✓	✓		✓	✓		X	X	✓	X	X	X	✓	✓	X	
SEP		X	X	✓		X	X	✓	✓		✓	✓	✓		✓	✓	✓	X	✓		✓	✓		X	X	X	X	X	X	
OCT				✓	✓	X	X	✓	✓							X		✓	X			X	X		X	X		✓			
NOV	✓	X			✓	✓	✓			✓	✓					✓				X							✓			
DEC					✓	✓	✓			✓	✓		X	X		✓			X	X	X					X				

	1	2	3	4	5	6	7	8	9	10	11	12	13	14	15	16	17	18	19	20	21	22	23	24	25	26	27	28	29	30	31
JAN																															
FEB																															
MAR																															
APR			✓	✓		✓	✓	✓	✓	✓	✓			✗	✗		✓		✗		✗	✗			✓	✓		✗		✓	
MAY			✓		✓	✗		✗	✓	✓	✗	✗		✗	✗			✗	✓			✓		✗							✓
JUN	✓				✗	✗	✗					✗	✓	✗	✗				✓		✗	✓	✓				✓	✓			
JUL		✓	✓	✓								✗	✗			✓	✓		✗				✓		✓	✓	✓	✓			
AUG	✗	✗	✓	✗				✗	✗		✗	✓	✓	✗	✗	✓	✓	✓	✓		✓	✓		✗	✗	✗	✓	✗	✗		
SEP				✗	✗					✓			✓		✓	✓	✓	✓	✓	✓	✓	✓			✗	✗					
OCT	✗	✗			✗				✗							✓							✗	✗	✗	✗			✗	✗	
NOV					✗	✓	✓	✓			✓	✓				✓	✗	✗	✗	✓	✓	✓	✗	✓	✓	✗					
DEC	✗	✗						✓	✓							✗	✗	✓	✓			✗	✗	✗	✗		✓	✓			

LIBRA 1990

1990	1	2	3	4	5	6	7	8	9	10	11	12	13	14	15	16	17	18	19	20	21	22	23	24	25	26	27	28	29	30	31
JAN																															
FEB																															
MAR																															
APR	✗	✗		✓		✓	✓		✓	✓					✓	✗	✗			✗			✗	✗					✗		
MAY	✓	✓	✓	✗							✓		✗	✗		✗				✗	✗		✗	✓		✗	✗				
JUN		✓	✓				✓	✓	✗	✗	✗	✓				✓							✗	✗		✓		✓		✓	
JUL						✓	✓	✓		✓	✗			✗	✗	✗	✓	✓			✗	✗	✓	✓			✓				
AUG	✓		✗			✗	✗			✗	✓	✓	✗	✓		✗	✗			✓	✗			✓						✗	✗
SEP	✗		✓	✓				✓		✗	✓			✗			✓	✓		✓	✓			✗	✗		✗	✗			✗
OCT			✗	✗	✓		✗	✓	✓	✗	✗		✓	✓	✗				✓		✗	✗		✗			✗	✗	✗		
NOV	✗				✓	✗	✗		✓	✓	✓	✓	✓	✓					✓		✗	✗			✗		✗	✗	✗		
DEC				✗	✗	✓				✓	✓	✓					✓	✗	✗						✗	✗					

SCORPIO

1990

	1	2	3	4	5	6	7	8	9	10	11	12	13	14	15	16	17	18	19	20	21	22	23	24	25	26	27	28	29	30	31
JAN																															
FEB																															
MAR																															
APR	✗	✗	✓	✓	✗		✓				✓	✓					✓	✗	✗	✗					✗	✗	✗			✓	
MAY	✓		✓					✓	✓	✓			✗			✗	✗		✗			✗	✗								✓
JUN		✓	✓		✓	✓						✓			✓					✗		✓			✗			✓			
JUL		✓	✓					✓		✗	✗	✓	✗			✗	✗		✗				✗	✓	✓					✓	✓
AUG			✓		✗	✗	✗	✓	✓			✗	✓			✓			✓	✗			✓			✓	✓				
SEP		✓	✓		✗			✗	✗			✓	✓	✗	✗	✗			✓	✓		✓	✓							✗	
OCT	✗	✓			✗	✗	✗	✗					✗		✓	✗			✓	✓							✗	✗	✓		
NOV		✗	✗			✓	✓	✗	✗			✓				✓					✓	✗	✗							✗	
DEC	✗			✓		✗							✓	✓					✗	✗		✗	✗				✗	✗			✓

1990

	1	2	3	4	5	6	7	8	9	10	11	12	13	14	15	16	17	18	19	20	21	22	23	24	25	26	27	28	29	30	31
JAN																															
FEB																															
MAR																											✗	✗			
APR					✓					✓	✓	✓			✓	✓					✗	✗		✗	✗		✗	✗			
MAY	✓	✓	✓																											✓	✗
JUN	✗					✓	✓	✓	✓					✗		✓		✗	✗		✓	✗		✗	✗	✓					
JUL					✓	✓			✗			✗	✗	✗	✗	✗		✓	✗		✗	✗				✓	✗				
AUG	✓	✓				✓								✗	✗				✗	✓		✗	✓			✗		✓	✓		
SEP			✓															✗	✗	✓		✗						✓	✓		
OCT		✗	✗	✓	✗			✗		✗	✗			✗	✗		✓	✓				✓	✓	✓	✓	✓			✗	✗	
NOV	✓			✗	✗			✓		✗	✗		✓					✓	✓								✗				
DEC		✗	✗		✓	✓		✗	✗	✓						✗	✗					✗	✗			✗			✗	✗	

	1	2	3	4	5	6	7	8	9	10	11	12	13	14	15	16	17	18	19	20	21	22	23	24	25	26	27	28	29	30	31
JAN																															
FEB																															
MAR																															
APR	✗	✗	✓	✓	✗	✓	✗	✓	✓	✗	✓							✓		✗	✗		✗	✗	✓	✓		✓	✗	✗	
MAY			✗	✓	✓	✗	✗	✓	✓	✓				✓	✓		✓	✓								✗	✗				
JUN	✓	✗	✓	✓	✓			✓		✓	✓			✗		✗	✗		✓	✗	✗	✗	✗	✗				✓			
JUL	✗	✓	✓	✓			✓	✓	✓	✗	✗			✗	✗	✗	✗			✗	✗	✓		✓	✓		✗	✗	✓		✓
AUG					✓			✓	✗	✗	✗	✗	✓	✗	✗	✗	✗			✗				✗			✓	✗			✗
SEP	✓		✓	✓	✓					✓					✓				✓	✓					✓		✓	✓			
OCT		✓		✗	✗	✗	✗		✗	✗	✗	✗	✗		✓	✗	✗	✗						✓	✓		✓		✓	✗	✗
NOV	✗	✓				✗	✗			✗		✓	✓	✗							✓	✓						✗	✗		
DEC				✗	✗						✗			✓				✓	✓			✓		✓		✗	✗	✓	✓		✗

AQUARIUS

1990

1990	1	2	3	4	5	6	7	8	9	10	11	12	13	14	15	16	17	18	19	20	21	22	23	24	25	26	27	28	29	30	31
JAN																															
FEB																															
MAR																															
APR	✓			✗	✗					✓	✓	✗			✓	✓	✓		✓	✓					✗	✗	✗				
MAY		✗	✗	✗	✗			✗	✗	✗	✓											✗	✗	✓	✗	✗		✗	✗		
JUN				✓			✓	✓			✓		✓				✓		✓	✗	✓				✗	✗					
JUL			✗	✓		✓				✓		✓	✗					✓	✗			✗	✗		✗	✗					✗
AUG	✓	✓				✓						✗	✗	✓	✗	✗	✗	✗	✗	✓	✓	✗	✗	✓	✗	✗		✓	✓	✗	✗
SEP		✓	✓	✓					✗	✗								✓										✓		✓	
OCT	✓			✓	✓	✗		✓	✓	✓	✓	✗	✗	✓	✗	✗	✓			✗	✗	✗	✗	✗							
NOV	✓	✓	✗		✓	✗	✗	✗	✗	✓	✓		✓	✓	✗	✗	✗		✓	✓	✓	✓	✓	✓						✗	
DEC	✗					✗	✗						✗				✓										✗	✗			

PISCES

1990

1990	1	2	3	4	5	6	7	8	9	10	11	12	13	14	15	16	17	18	19	20	21	22	23	24	25	26	27	28	29	30	31
JAN	x																														
FEB																															
MAR																															
APR			x	x		x	x				✓		x	x			✓					✓			✓	✓✓	x	x		✓	
MAY		✓	✓	x	x			✓			x	x	x	✓					✓			✓		x	x						x
JUN		✓	✓		x		x	x			✓				✓	✓			✓		x					x	x	x			
JUL		✓✓	✓						✓			✓	✓		✓	✓		x	x					x	x	x	x			✓	✓
AUG	x			✓		✓		✓✓	x	✓	x	x	✓	x	x	✓	x	x	✓		x	x		x			✓	x	x	✓	
SEP						✓				✓			✓				x							x			✓				
OCT		✓✓				✓	✓				✓					✓	✓					✓	x	✓	✓	✓			✓	✓	
NOV		✓			x	✓	✓		x	x	x	x		✓	✓	✓	✓	x	x		✓			x	x	✓	✓			x	✓
DEC		x	x	✓				x	x					✓	✓		x		✓					✓					x	x	✓

ARIES

1991

1991	1	2	3	4	5	6	7	8	9	10	11	12	13	14	15	16	17	18	19	20	21	22	23	24	25	26	27	28	29	30	31
JAN	X	✓	✓			X	X	X			✓			X	X						✓	✓					X	X		✓	✓
FEB			X	X				✓	✓	X	X	X		✓				✓	✓			✓		X	X	✓					
MAR			X				✓	✓	X	X	✓	✓	✓				✓	✓				✓	X	X	✓	✓				X	X
APR		✓	✓	✓		X	X	✓					✓	✓			X	X	X	X		✓	✓	X		X	X	✓	✓	X	
MAY	✓	✓	✓	X	X	✓					✓	✓	✓	X	✓	X	X	X	X	✓	X	✓	X	X				✓	✓		
JUN	X		✓		✓	✓	✓	✓	✓	X	✓	✓	X	X			X	X	X	X	X		✓	✓	✓	✓		X			
JUL	✓				✓						✓	✓		✓		X	X		✓			✓	✓	✓	X	✓		✓	✓	X	✓
AUG	✓	✓			✓	✓		X	X	X	X		X	X				X	✓		X			✓	✓			✓	✓	X	
SEP			X	X		✓	X	X		X	✓	X	✓	✓	X	✓		✓	✓		✓	✓		✓	✓	✓	✓	✓	X	X	
OCT	X		✓	✓				X		X	✓	X			X	✓						✓		X	X	✓	✓	✓	✓	✓	
NOV			X	X				✓	✓	X	X	X	✓					✓	✓					X	X	✓	✓	X	X	X	
DEC	X	X			✓	✓		X			✓	X				✓	✓					X	X					X	X		

TAURUS

1991	1	2	3	4	5	6	7	8	9	10	11	12	13	14	15	16	17	18	19	20	21	22	23	24	25	26	27	28	29	30	31
JAN	✓	✗	✗	✓					✗	✗				✓	✓			✗						✓	✓					✗	✗
FEB	✓				✗	✗					✓	✓		✗		✓				✓	✓				✓	✗	✗	✗			
MAR		✗		✗	✗	✗					✓				✓	✓		✓	✓	✓	✗				✗	✗	✓	✓			
APR	✗	✗								✗	✓				✓	✓					✗	✗	✗	✓	✓	✗	✓	✗	✗		
MAY			✓		✗	✗		✓			✓		✓	✓			✓		✗	✗	✓	✗	✗		✗	✗	✗	✗		✓	✓
JUN		✓	✗		✓	✓	✓		✓	✓			✓		✗	✓	✓	✓				✓	✗	✓	✗		✓		✗	✗	
JUL							✓				✓	✗	✗		✗	✗	✗		✗	✗		✗		✓	✓	✗	✗	✗	✓	✗	
AUG		✓	✓	✓					✗	✗		✓			✗	✗	✓	✓		✓	✓		✗	✗			✓	✗	✓	✓	✓
SEP			✓	✗	✗	✗			✗	✗		✗	✗	✗		✗	✗			✗			✓	✓		✓	✓	✗	✓		
OCT	✓		✗	✗						✗				✓	✓		✗							✓	✓			✓		✗	✗
NOV	✓	✓	✗	✗	✗	✗	✗				✓	✓		✗						✓	✓				✓	✗	✗	✓			
DEC		✓	✗	✗			✗		✓		✗						✓	✓			✓			✗	✗		✓	✓		✗	✗

GEMINI 1991

1991	1	2	3	4	5	6	7	8	9	10	11	12	13	14	15	16	17	18	19	20	21	22	23	24	25	26	27	28	29	30	31
JAN		✓		✗	✗		✓	✓	✗			✗	✗			✓	✓		✗	✗						✓					✓
FEB	✗	✗			✓		✗	✗	✗				✓	✓		✗	✗	✓	✓			✓	✓					✗			
MAR	✗						✗	✗				✓	✓	✓	✗	✗	✗	✓			✓	✓			✓	✓		✗	✗		
APR			✗	✗	✗		✓	✓	✓			✗					✓	✓						✗	✗					✗	
MAY	✗	✗				✓									✓	✓				✓	✗	✓	✓	✓				✗	✗	✗	
JUN		✗	✓			✗	✓	✓	✓		✓	✓							✓	✓	✗	✗	✓	✓	✗	✗					
JUL	✓	✗			✓	✓	✓	✓		✗	✗	✗	✓	✗	✗		✗	✗	✗		✗	✗	✗	✗	✗	✗					
AUG	✓				✓	✓	✓	✓	✓	✓	✗	✗	✓	✗		✗	✗	✗	✗		✗	✗	✗	✓	✗	✗					
SEP	✓	✓										✗	✗		✗	✓	✓				✗	✗		✓		✓	✓	✓	✓	✗	
OCT			✓	✓	✗	✗	✓	✓	✗		✗	✗	✗		✗				✗	✗	✓						✓				
NOV	✗	✗		✓				✗	✗				✓	✓	✗	✗			✓		✗	✓	✓		✗		✓	✗	✗		
DEC		✓				✗					✓	✓	✗	✗		✓			✓							✗	✗				

1991	1	2	3	4	5	6	7	8	9	10	11	12	13	14	15	16	17	18	19	20	21	22	23	24	25	26	27	28	29	30	31
JAN	✓					✗	✗	✗		✓				✗	✗							✗	✓				✓	✓			
FEB			✗	✗		✓	✓			✗	✗	✗						✗		✓				✓	✓			✓			
MAR		✗	✗	✓	✓				✗	✗	✗			✓	✓	✓			✓				✓	✓					✗	✗	✗
APR	✓	✓		✓			✗		✓		✓	✓	✗	✗	✓		✓	✓	✓	✓			✓	✓		✗	✗	✓	✓	✓	✓
MAY			✗	✓	✗	✓	✗	✗	✓		✗	✗	✓				✓	✓			✓	✓	✗	✗			✓		✓	✗	✗
JUN	✗	✗		✗	✓	✓	✗			✓			✓	✓			✗	✗		✗	✗						✗	✗			
JUL		✓	✓				✓	✓		✓	✓	✓			✓	✓			✓												
AUG		✗		✓			✓	✓	✗	✗		✓	✗	✗	✓	✗	✗	✗		✗	✗	✗		✗	✗						
SEP			✓	✓								✓	✓	✗	✗								✓		✗	✓	✓		✗	✓	
OCT	✓						✓		✓	✓					✓					✓		✗		✓	✓	✓	✓	✓	✓		
NOV			✗	✗		✓	✓			✗	✗	✗						✗		✓	✓				✓						
DEC	✗	✗	✓	✓			✗	✗	✗				✓				✗	✓			✓	✓						✗	✗	✓	

	1	2	3	4	5	6	7	8	9	10	11	12	13	14	15	16	17	18	19	20	21	22	23	24	25	26	27	28	29	30	31
JAN	✓			✓	✓					✓		✗	✗	✓	✓				✗	✗			✓	✓		✗	✗				
FEB	✓	✓	✓				✓	✗	✗		✓	✓			✗	✗				✓		✗	✗			✓		✓			
MAR	✓						✗	✗			✓	✓		✗	✗	✗		✓	✓	✓		✗						✓	✓		
APR	✓		✓	✗	✗						✗	✗	✓		✓	✓	✗	✗						✓	✓				✓	✗	
MAY	✗	✗		✗	✗	✗		✗	✗				✓			✗						✓			✗	✗	✓	✗	✓	✓	✓
JUN		✗	✗	✗	✗				✗	✓	✗	✗	✓	✓	✓		✓	✓			✓	✓			✗		✓	✓	✗	✓	
JUL		✗									✓			✓	✓								✗	✓	✗	✗	✓	✓	✗	✗	
AUG					✗		✓	✓	✓		✓	✓		✗	✗		✓	✗		✓	✓	✗	✗		✓	✗		✗	✗	✗	
SEP	✗	✗	✓				✓	✓	✓			✓		✓	✗											✓	✓	✗	✗		
OCT	✓	✓			✓	✓		✗	✗			✗			✓		✗		✗	✗		✗	✗	✓		✗	✗	✓	✓		
NOV	✓	✓				✓			✗		✓				✗	✗				✓		✗	✓		✓			✓	✓		
DEC			✓		✗	✗	✗		✓				✗	✗				✓	✓	✗	✗		✗				✓				

LEO

1991

1991	1	2	3	4	5	6	7	8	9	10	11	12	13	14	15	16	17	18	19	20	21	22	23	24	25	26	27	28	29	30	31
JAN		✓	✓						✗	✗	✓						✗	✗			✓	✓		✗	✗					✓	✓
FEB					✗	✗	✗	✓	✓				✗	✗				✓	✓	✗	✗					✓	✓				
MAR				✓	✗	✗	✓	✓				✗	✗					✓	✗	✗	✓	✓	✓		✓	✓					
APR	✗	✗	✓					✗	✗	✗					✓		✓											✗	✗		
MAY	✓	✓	✗			✗	✓		✗	✓			✗	✗	✓	✓		✓	✓	✓					✗	✗	✗	✓	✓		
JUN		✗	✗		✓				✗		✓	✓			✓	✓			✓			✗	✗	✓					✗	✗	
JUL	✗											✓	✓			✓	✓			✗		✓	✓	✗		✗	✗	✗	✗		✓
AUG	✓	✓	✗	✗	✓	✓	✓		✓	✓		✓	✓	✓		✗	✗	✗	✗	✗				✗	✓			✓		✗	✗
SEP						✓			✗	✗		✗	✗	✓					✗	✗				✓	✗		✗				
OCT		✓		✓	✓	✓	✗		✗	✗		✓	✗					✗	✗	✓	✓										
NOV				✓		✗	✗	✓					✗	✗		✓	✓	✓	✓							✓	✓			✓	✓
DEC		✓	✗	✗	✓	✓				✗	✗					✓	✓	✗	✗											✗	✗

LIBRA

1991

1991	1	2	3	4	5	6	7	8	9	10	11	12	13	14	15	16	17	18	19	20	21	22	23	24	25	26	27	28	29	30	31
JAN	✗	✓	✓				✓	✓						✗	✗	✓	✓				✗	✗						✗	✗		
FEB		✓	✓	✓							✗	✗	✓	✓	✓		✗	✗						✗		✓					
MAR		✓	✓				✓			✗	✗	✓	✓			✗	✗	✗					✗	✗						✓	✓
APR			✓			✗	✗						✗				✓	✓	✗	✗		✓				✓	✓				
MAY	✓				✗	✓	✓	✗	✓	✗		✗			✓	✓	✗	✗	✗	✗		✓	✓	✓	✗			✓			✗
JUN	✗		✓	✗	✗			✗	✓	✗	✓	✓		✗						✓	✓		✓	✓	✗		✗	✗			
JUL	✓						✗	✗			✗							✓	✓	✓	✓	✓	✓	✗	✗	✓					✗
AUG	✗				✓	✓	✓	✗	✓	✓			✓	✓	✗	✓	✗	✗	✓	✓	✗	✗	✓	✗	✗		✗	✗	✗		
SEP		✓					✓	✓		✓	✗		✓	✗	✗	✓	✗													✓	
OCT	✗	✗	✓	✓	✓		✓	✓			✗	✗		✗			✗	✗	✗		✗	✗		✗	✗				✗		
NOV		✓	✓	✓					✗		✗	✗		✓		✓	✓	✗	✗			✓		✗			✓			✓	
DEC	✓	✓			✓			✗	✗		✓	✓			✗	✗						✗	✗								

	1	2	3	4	5	6	7	8	9	10	11	12	13	14	15	16	17	18	19	20	21	22	23	24	25	26	27	28	29	30	31
JAN	✓		✗						✓	✓								✗	✓					✗	✗			✓	✓	✓	✗
FEB					✓	✓	✗				✓		✗	✗	✗			✗	✗	✗	✗			✓	✓	✓		✗			
MAR					✓	✓					✓	✗	✗	✓	✓	✓			✗	✗					✗			✓			
APR	✓	✓							✗	✗	✓	✓			✗	✗					✗							✓	✓		
MAY				✓	✓	✗	✗	✓	✓			✗	✗	✗		✗	✓		✗		✓						✓			✓	
JUN		✗	✗	✗		✓	✗		✗	✗	✓	✓	✓	✓	✓	✗	✓					✓	✓			✓			✗	✗	
JUL		✓	✓	✓			✓	✓	✗	✗	✓	✓	✓			✓	✓	✓	✓	✓				✓			✗	✗	✓	✓	
AUG		✗	✓	✓				✓	✓	✓		✓	✓				✗	✗	✗	✗			✗	✗		✗	✗			✗	✗
SEP			✓	✗		✗								✗					✗				✗			✗	✗			✓	
OCT	✓						✓		✓	✓	✓		✓	✓	✓					✗	✗				✗			✓	✓		
NOV											✓		✗	✗	✓			✗	✗	✗	✗				✓			✓			
DEC			✓	✓					✓	✗	✗		✓				✗	✗						✗	✗					✓	

SAGITTARIUS

1991	1	2	3	4	5	6	7	8	9	10	11	12	13	14	15	16	17	18	19	20	21	22	23	24	25	26	27	28	29	30	31
JAN		✓	✓	✗	✗							✓	✓						✗	✗	✓	✓				✗				✓	✓
FEB	✗	✗		✓				✓	✓					✓	✗	✗		✓	✓			✗	✗					✓			
MAR	✗						✓	✓	✓				✓		✗	✗		✓			✗	✗			✓	✓				✓	
APR				✓	✓	✗		✓	✗	✓	✗	✗			✗		✗	✗			✗			✗	✗						
MAY	✓	✓				✓	✓	✗	✗		✗	✗			✗	✗				✓	✓	✗	✓		✓	✓		✓	✓	✓	
JUN			✓			✗	✓		✗	✓	✗	✗			✗			✗	✓				✓		✓	✓					
JUL	✓	✗								✗			✓				✓		✓			✓	✓						✗	✗	
AUG	✓	✓			✓	✓	✓	✗		✗	✗	✓			✓			✓	✓						✗	✗		✓	✗	✗	
SEP	✗	✗		✓	✗	✗	✗	✗		✗			✓			✓	✓		✗	✗	✗	✗	✗	✓	✗	✗	✗	✗	✗	✗	
OCT			✓	✓	✓			✓	✓			✓	✓	✓		✓	✓	✓	✓		✓	✓		✓	✓	✗	✓			✓	
NOV	✗	✗		✓		✓							✓			✗	✗		✓			✗	✗			✓	✓	✗	✗		
DEC	✓	✓			✓	✓					✓		✗	✗		✓	✓			✗	✗					✗	✗				

1991

	1	2	3	4	5	6	7	8	9	10	11	12	13	14	15	16	17	18	19	20	21	22	23	24	25	26	27	28	29	30	31
JAN	✗			✓		✗								✓	✓						✗	✗	✓	✓			✗	✗			
FEB	✓		✗	✗		✓	✓				✓	✓		✓	✓			✗	✗	✓	✓			✗	✗		✗				
MAR		✗	✗	✗		✓	✓			✓	✓	✓	✗	✗			✗	✗	✗	✓	✓		✗	✗	✗			✓		✗	✗
APR	✓					✓	✓						✗	✗	✓	✓	✓	✗	✗	✗			✗	✓	✓	✗	✗				
MAY				✓	✓			✓	✗	✗	✗	✗	✓	✓	✓	✓	✗	✗			✓	✓					✓	✓		✓	✓
JUN	✓			✓	✓		✓		✗	✓		✗	✗	✗	✓	✓	✓	✓		✗	✓	✓				✗	✓	✓			
JUL	✗	✓			✗			✗		✗	✗		✗	✗	✓	✓	✗				✓			✓	✓		✓	✓	✓		✗
AUG	✗						✗	✗	✗	✗	✗	✓		✓	✓	✓	✓	✓		✓	✓	✓	✓	✓	✗		✓	✗	✗		
SEP			✗	✗				✗	✗	✗	✗	✓		✓	✓		✓	✓				✗	✓	✗	✗	✓	✓	✗	✗	✗	
OCT	✗							✗	✓	✗	✓	✓		✓	✓			✗	✗	✗	✓	✗	✓	✓	✗		✓	✗	✗		✗
NOV	✓		✗			✓		✗	✗		✓	✓					✗	✗	✗	✓	✓	✗	✓	✗	✗		✗	✓	✗	✗	
DEC	✗	✗	✓					✓	✓						✗	✗	✗	✓	✓		✗	✗	✗				✓	✗	✗		

AQUARIUS

1991	1	2	3	4	5	6	7	8	9	10	11	12	13	14	15	16	17	18	19	20	21	22	23	24	25	26	27	28	29	30	31
JAN		✗	✗				✓	✓	✗	✗														✗	✗					✗	✗
FEB					✓	✓	✗				✓		✓	✓				✓		✗	✗	✓				✗	✗				
MAR				✓		✗	✓					✓	✓					✓	✗	✗	✓		✗			✗					
APR			✓	✓					✓	✓					✗	✗		✓					✓		✗			✗			
MAY	✓					✓	✓						✗	✗	✓	✓			✗	✗		✗	✓	✓	✗	✗		✓			
JUN		✓	✓		✓	✓			✗	✗	✓	✓				✗	✓		✓	✓		✓		✓					✓	✓	
JUL	✓				✓	✓	✗		✗	✗	✓	✗	✗		✗	✗	✓	✓		✗			✓					✓			
AUG	✓	✓	✗	✗	✓	✓		✓	✓	✓			✓	✓		✗	✗	✓	✓					✓	✗	✗				✗	✗
SEP		✓			✗	✗				✗		✗													✓	✗	✗				
OCT			✗	✗			✓	✓	✓	✗					✓		✓	✓	✓	✓				✗	✓	✗	✗			✗	✗
NOV				✓		✗	✗						✓	✓				✓	✓	✗	✗	✓				✗	✗			✗	
DEC		✓		✗	✓	✓					✓	✓				✓	✓	✗					✗	✗		✗				✗	✗

PISCES

1991

1991	1	2	3	4	5	6	7	8	9	10	11	12	13	14	15	16	17	18	19	20	21	22	23	24	25	26	27	28	29	30	31
JAN	✓			✗	✗					✓	✗	✗	✗		✓				✓	✓						✗		✓			
FEB	✗	✗	✗			✓	✓		✗	✗	✓				✓	✓						✗	✗		✓	✓		✗			
MAR	✗			✓	✓	✓	✗	✗						✓	✓	✓	✗	✗			✗	✗		✗			✗	✗	✗		
APR	✓	✓		✗	✗			✗			✓	✓					✓				✗	✓	✓	✗			✓		✓	✓	
MAY	✗	✗				✓			✓				✓	✓	✗		✗	✗			✗				✗	✗	✓			✓	
JUN		✓	✓			✓				✓	✓	✓	✓	✓							✗		✗	✓		✗					
JUL			✓	✓											✗				✓					✓					✓	✓	
AUG				✓		✗	✓	✗	✗		✗	✗		✗	✓	✗		✗		✓					✓	✓					
SEP	✗	✗			✗	✗	✗	✗	✓	✓	✗	✗	✓	✗	✗	✗	✓	✓	✓	✓		✓	✓			✓	✗	✗		✓	
OCT	✓					✗			✓	✓	✓		✗	✓	✓	✓	✓		✓	✓				✓	✗	✗	✗	✓			
NOV	✗	✗				✓	✓	✗	✗		✓		✓	✓		✓				✓		✗	✗		✓			✗	✗		
DEC				✓	✗	✗	✗		✓			✓	✓	✓				✓	✗	✗	✗					✗	✗				

ARIES

1992	1	2	3	4	5	6	7	8	9	10	11	12	13	14	15	16	17	18	19	20	21	22	23	24	25	26	27	28	29	30	31
JAN	✓	✓		✗	✗	✓					✓	✓	✓			✓		✗	✗	✓	✓			✗	✗				✓	✓	✗
FEB	✗		✓	✓				✓	✓			✓		✗	✗		✓			✗	✗				✓	✓		✗	✗		
MAR		✓				✓	✓				✓		✗	✗		✓			✗	✗			✓	✓			✗				
APR																															
MAY																															
JUN																															
JUL																															
AUG																															
SEP																															
OCT																															
NOV																															
DEC																															

1992

TAURUS

1992

1992	1	2	3	4	5	6	7	8	9	10	11	12	13	14	15	16	17	18	19	20	21	22	23	24	25	26	27	28	29	30	31
JAN				✓	✓		✗		✓					✓	✓					✗	✗	✓	✓			✗	✗				✓
FEB		✗	✗	✗	✓	✓		✓		✓	✓					✗	✗	✓	✓			✗	✗	✗			✓	✓			
MAR	✗			✓				✓	✓						✗	✗	✓	✓			✗	✗			✗	✗		✗	✗		
APR																															
MAY																															
JUN																															
JUL																															
AUG																															
SEP																															
OCT																															
NOV																															
DEC																															

GEMINI

1992

1992	1	2	3	4	5	6	7	8	9	10	11	12	13	14	15	16	17	18	19	20	21	22	23	24	25	26	27	28	29	30	31
JAN	X	X	X			✓	✓	✓		X						✓	✓			✓		X	X	✓				X	X	X	
FEB			✓	✓	X	X						✓	✓				✓	X	X		✓				X	X					
MAR		✓	X	X		✓				✓	✓	✓					X	X	✓	✓			X	X				✓			
APR																															
MAY																															
JUN																															
JUL																															
AUG																															
SEP																															
OCT																															
NOV																															
DEC																															

CANCER — 1992

	1	2	3	4	5	6	7	8	9	10	11	12	13	14	15	16	17	18	19	20	21	22	23	24	25	26	27	28	29	30	31
JAN				x	x				✓	✓	x	x		✓				✓	✓			✓		x	x						x
FEB	x		✓		✓	✓		x	x	✓				✓	✓				✓	x	x			✓			x	x	x		
MAR			✓	✓	✓	x	x		✓				✓	✓			✓	✓	x	x					x	x	x				
APR																															
MAY																															
JUN																															
JUL																															
AUG																															
SEP																															
OCT																															
NOV																															
DEC																															

	1	2	3	4	5	6	7	8	9	10	11	12	13	14	15	16	17	18	19	20	21	22	23	24	25	26	27	28	29	30	31
JAN	✓	✓				✗	✗	✗							✗	✓	✓			✓	✓					✗	✗		✓	✓	
FEB		✗	✗	✗						✗	✗	✓				✓	✓					✗	✗	✗	✓	✓					
MAR	✗	✗				✓	✗				✓				✓	✓			✓		✗	✗						✗	✗		
APR																															
MAY																															
JUN																															
JUL																															
AUG																															
SEP																															
OCT																															
NOV																															
DEC																															

VIRGO

1992

	1	2	3	4	5	6	7	8	9	10	11	12	13	14	15	16	17	18	19	20	21	22	23	24	25	26	27	28	29	30	31
JAN	x	x	x x	✓	✓	✓			x	x				✓	✓	✓ x	x					✓	✓						x	x	✓
FEB					x	x				✓	✓		x					✓	✓						x	x x	✓	✓			
MAR			x	x	x				✓	✓ ✓	x						✓	✓					x	x	✓	✓				x	x
APR																															
MAY																															
JUN																															
JUL																															
AUG																															
SEP																															
OCT																															
NOV																															
DEC																															

LIBRA

1992	1	2	3	4	5	6	7	8	9	10	11	12	13	14	15	16	17	18	19	20	21	22	23	24	25	26	27	28	29	30	31
JAN	✓			✗	✗	✓	✓				✗	✗	✗			✓		✗	✗	✓				✓	✓				✓		✗
FEB	✗		✓	✓			✗	✗	✗			✓	✓	✗	✗		✓			✓	✓						✗	✗	✗		
MAR		✓				✗	✗				✓	✓	✗	✗					✓	✓			✓			✗	✗	✓			
APR																															
MAY																															
JUN																															
JUL																															
AUG																															
SEP																															
OCT																															
NOV																															
DEC																															

SCORPIO 1992

1992	1	2	3	4	5	6	7	8	9	10	11	12	13	14	15	16	17	18	19	20	21	22	23	24	25	26	27	28	29	30	31
JAN		x		✓	✓	x	x	x	✓	✓			x	x	x					x		✓				✓	✓				✓
FEB			x	x	✓	✓				x	x			✓		x			✓				x	x			x				
MAR	x	x	✓	✓	✓			x	x				✓		x		✓	✓			✓	✓						x	x		
APR																															
MAY																															
JUN																															
JUL																															
AUG																															
SEP																															
OCT																															
NOV																															
DEC																															

	1	2	3	4	5	6	7	8	9	10	11	12	13	14	15	16	17	18	19	20	21	22	23	24	25	26	27	28	29	30	31
JAN	✓	✓	✓			✓	✓		✗	✗						✗	✗			✓	✓	✗	✗						✓	✓	
FEB			✓		✗	✗						✗	✗				✓		✗						✓	✓					
MAR		✓	✗	✗	✗	✓				✗	✗					✓		✗	✓				✓	✓				✓			
APR																															
MAY																															
JUN																															
JUL																															
AUG																															
SEP																															
OCT																															
NOV																															
DEC																															

	1	2	3	4	5	6	7	8	9	10	11	12	13	14	15	16	17	18	19	20	21	22	23	24	25	26	27	28	29	30	31
JAN				✓	✓				✓		✗	✗	✗	✓	✓			✗	✗			✓	✓	✗	✗						✓
FEB					✓	✓	✗	✗	✗	✓	✓			✗	✗			✓	✓		✗						✓	✓	✓		
MAR				✓		✗	✗		✓	✓		✗	✗	✗			✓	✓		✗						✓	✓				
APR																															
MAY																															
JUN																															
JUL																															
AUG																															
SEP																															
OCT																															
NOV																															
DEC																															

1992	1	2	3	4	5	6	7	8	9	10	11	12	13	14	15	16	17	18	19	20	21	22	23	24	25	26	27	28	29	30	31
JAN	✓					✓	✓	✓						x	x	✓								✓		x	x		✓		
FEB		✓	✓	✓	✓					x	x	✓	✓							✓	✓	x	x		✓						
MAR	✓	✓						x	x		✓	✓			x	x	x		✓	✓	x	x						✓	✓		
APR																															
MAY																															
JUN																															
JUL																															
AUG																															
SEP																															
OCT																															
NOV																															
DEC																															

PISCES

1992	1	2	3	4	5	6	7	8	9	10	11	12	13	14	15	16	17	18	19	20	21	22	23	24	25	26	27	28	29	30	31
JAN	x	x		✓					✓	✓				✓		x	x					x	x	✓		x				x	✓
FEB					✓	✓				✓		x	x	✓				x	x								✓	✓			
MAR			✓	✓	✓				✓	x	x	x	✓				x	x								✓					✓
APR																															
MAY																															
JUN																															
JUL																															
AUG																															
SEP																															
OCT																															
NOV																															
DEC